Scientific Insights in Yoga

Scientific Insights in Yoga

Dr. Shashi Bala Singh

Dr. K.P. Mishra

Foreword

Dr. Nagendra

PRABHAT PRAKASHAN

ISO 9001: 2008 Publishers

Published by
PRABHAT PRAKASHAN
4/19 Asaf Ali Road,
New Delhi-110 002 (INDIA)
Tele : +91-11-23289777
e-mail: prabhatbooks@gmail.com

ISBN 978-93-5266-899-1
SCIENTIFIC INSIGHTS IN YOGA
by Dr. Shashi Bala Singh
Dr. K.P. Mishra

Edition
First, 2018

Price
₹ 450.00 (Rupees Four Hundred Fifty only)

Printed at
R-Tech Offset Printers, Delhi

This book is dedicated to
the people who practice yoga
for promoting health and
preventing diseases

स्वामी विवेकानन्द योग अनुसंधान संस्थान
Swami Vivekananda Yoga Anusandhāna Samsthāna
(Declared as Deemed-to-be University under Section 3 of the UGC Act, 1956)
Eknath Bhavan, # 19, Gavipuram Circle, Kempegowda Nagar, Bangalore - 560 019
Ph: 080 - 2661 2669, Telefax: 080 - 2660 8645
E-mail: svyasa@svyasa.org Website: www.svyasa.org

Foreword

The origins of yoga have been speculated to date back to pre-vedic Indian traditions, as mentioned in the Rigveda. The ancient wisdom known as "the supreme science of life" is believed to have been revealed to the great sages of India several thousand years ago. The first written records of the practice of yoga appeared around 200 BC in *Yogasutra* of Patanjali. The system consisted of the eightfold path or *Asthangayoga*. Yoga is a union of the organ systems in the body with the consciousness in the mind. Philosophically, yoga produces a union of body, mind, soul or spirit, to bring about a state of equanimity (calmness). Progressing to an even more advanced state, blending science and philosophy, one experiences a union of body, mind, internal energy, and all-pervading cosmic energy, resulting in better physical health, mental control, and ultimately self-realization. Yoga is a systematic practice of physical exercise, breath control, realization, positive thinking and meditation aimed at developing harmony in the body, mind, and environment. The practice entails low-impact physical activity, postures (called *asanas*), breathing techniques (*pranayama*), relaxation, and meditation. Yoga is not a thing merely to be heard. Yoga is a thing that has to be assimilated and put into practice in daily life. Yoga does not quarrel with science; it supplements it. Yoga is an exact comprehensive science that helps to control and co-ordinate the subtle forces within the body. Through yoga we can also have increased energy, vigour, vitality, longevity and a high standard of health. It removes fatigue, confers serenity, calmness, and wonderful concentration. Yoga is the science that teaches us the most effective way, how to remove our defects and weaknesses, and how to attain the state of perfection, freedom and superconscious blessedness. The state in which there is union with the absolute.

The present book entitled "Scientific Insights in Yoga" is a well-prepared and comprehensive book with updated scientific information. It is divided into three sections. Section 1: "Yoga as a Preventive Medicine", Section 2: "Yoga for Extreme Environments" and 3rd section consists of "Yoga as a Non-pharmacological Intervention in Diseases". The book will make the readers acquainted with the current researches and developments in this field. The chapters on yoga for extreme environments such as high altitude, extreme cold, hot deserts and submarine environment are very useful for the readers and those who are living in such environment. I am sure this book will add new dimensions to the research in non-pharmacological preventive medicine.

With Love,

(Dr. H.R. Nagendra)
Chancellor

Preface

The book "Scientific Insights in Yoga" introduces a range of perspectives in the field of yoga as a non-pharmacological intervention for promoting health under extremes of environmental conditions and disease stress. Special attention has been given to research leading to improvement of health of people living in extremes of environment. It serves as a guide as well as a reference book for practicing clinicians, scientists, and research scholars.

This book is divided into three sections: Section I: "Yoga as a Preventive Medicine", Section II: "Yoga for Extreme Environment" and Section III: "Yoga as a Non-pharmacological Intervention in Diseases".

Under the part I, different forms and styles of yoga; physiological basis of asana and pranayama; effects of yoga and meditation on mind-body health; stress management through yoga and effectiveness of yoga on physical performance and well-being has been broughtout.

Part two highlights the different yogic practices for extreme environmental conditions. Stay in extremely hostile environment such as desert, high altitude, confined environment and extreme cold areas etc. lead to detrimental physiological effects. How the different yogasanas and prananyama promote health and prevent detrimental effects of hostile environments are clearly described.

Part three covers the scientific validation of effects of yoga on different diseases such as asthma, obesity and eating disorder, sleep apnea, ageing related problems; cardiovascular diseases; diabetes; osteoporosis; rheumatoid arthritis and impaired neurocognition.

The authors has endeavored to present the text of this book in an interesting manner. Overall this book brings important scientific studies on yoga for preventing diseases and promoting health performance even in extreme of environmental conditions and disease stress.

Contents

Section III : Yoga as a Non-pharmacological Intervention in Diseases

Section I

Yoga as a Preventive Medicine

1
Different Forms and Styles of Yoga

Yoga is basically a type of exercise that affects not only the muscles of the body but also the function of the internal organs as well as the mental condition of a person. These exercises were practiced in ancient India more than 5000 years ago by sages. Yoga, besides being an excellent method of exercise is a meditation form as well.

History of Yoga

Yoga is the ancient wisdom originated in India thousands of years ago. It is a panacea for happiness and alleviation from all kind of sufferings. Lord Shiva is considered as the founder of Yoga. Evidences in the form of seals and fossil are obtained from the Indus Valley Civilisation dating back to 2700 BC which indicated the prevalence of yoga in ancient India. However, the first evidence of Yoga was described in the literature by Maharishi Patanjali in his Book *Yogdarshana*. Maharishi Patanjali has systematized yoga and its many postures. With the passage of time, other sages and yogis contributed in its development. Today, yoga is spread all over the world. On 11 December 2014, the United Nations General Assembly along with 193 members approved the proposal of Indian Prime Minister Sri Narendra Modi to celebrate the 21st of June as 'International Yoga Day'.

There are six principle types of yoga each offering different benefits; each could be used separately or in unison. The six different types of yoga are explained here:

The forms of Yoga

1. Hatha Yoga: This is the most common form of yoga practiced today. The meaning of 'Ha' is 'sun' and 'tha' means moon. Hatha yoga brings together the energy of the sun and the moon towards a complete balance in the body. This type of yoga is considered as a great method of physical therapy. Hatha yoga uses different postures combined with breathing exercises to purify both body and mind and thereby controlling and reversing a number of diseases.

The most prevalent tradition of yoga is Hatha Yoga. It basically involves eight steps: Yama, Niyama, Asana, Pranayama, Pratyahara, Dharana, Dhyana and Samadhi.

- **Yama and Niyama:** These are initial sets of principles that are concerned with our conduct in personal and social life. These are related to ethics and values.

  Yama: It consists of: –
  - a) Ahinsa (Nonviolence)
  - b) Satya (Truth)
  - c) Asteya (Non-stealing)
  - d) Brahamacharya (Celibacy)
  - e) Aparigraha (non-hoarding)

  Niyama
  - a) Shaucha (Internal cleanliness of body)
  - b) Santosha (Contentment)
  - c) Tap
  - d) Svadhyaya (Study of the self)
  - e) Ishvara Pranidhana (Dedication to the lord)
- **Asana:** Asanas are a series of postures, which brings flexibility, strength and balance in the body for greater health and well-being. These asanas are practiced for variable time periods depending on the practitioner's experience and the style of yoga he/she follows. These asanas require guidance and special attention by a qualified yoga teacher.
- **Pranayama:** Pranayama are breathing techniques. It is an integral part of many yoga styles. Throughout yoga practice, movement should be connected with the breath. In some postures, inhale is associated with one direction and exhale is associated with opposite direction. Some yoga gurus also teach to hold a posture

for a particular number of breaths. Some yoga teachers teach the breathing practices after asanas such as kapalbhati, anulom-vilom, bhasrika, ujjayi to calm the body and mind, these breathing techniques should be practiced with qualified yoga teacher.

- **Pratyahara:** Yogic practice of pratyahara means withdrawal of senses from sense organs in order to control mind. In pratyahara, the awareness about the external surrounding is withdrawn and is taken to inside. Introspection can help in pratyahara.
- **Dharana:** It refers to concentration of the mind. Practicing dharana involves fixing the mind on a particular object — either external (such as an image or deity) or internal (such as a chakra). Yoga can help an individual master the art of dharana because it involves focusing on the breath, body or even a mantra. Regular practice of dharana enhances yoga practice by improving the practitioner's ability to remain focused, no matter what they are doing. It trains the mind to remain calm and increases mental strength.
- **Dhyana:** Dhyana or meditation is the state of deep concentration, calmness and tranquility of the mind. It is the state of attaining complete control over one's mind. Meditation takes the consciousness beyond conscious, sub conscious & unconscious states to super consciousness. During meditation one should be quiet and focus the mind and free from trivial thoughts. It allows greater spiritual awakening and provides relief from stresses. During meditation, one can focus on anything such as the breath, an image, an idea, a sound, or a personal prayer. During meditation, traditional padmasana pose may be followed but can be done by sitting on chair as well.
- **Samadhi:** Samadhi is derived from the Sanskrit, sama, meaning together, and dhi, meaning mind. Its most basic definition implies a complete state of concentration. For a practitioner of yoga and for a disciple of meditation, the spiritual significance of samadhi is much more profound. Simply stated, samadhi is the mind's ultimate state of being; it is enlightenment and the preliminary state to nirvana.

Hatha Yoga has been passed from many gurus (teachers) to many shishya (students). Today, there are many styles of Hatha yoga which have different methods of practice.

Various styles of hatha yoga are described below

Anand: The founder of this style of hatha yoga is Swami Kriyananda. This style of yoga is very gentle. It prepares body for meditation and energizing the individual. Ananda Yoga, intended to improve the flow of energy through the chakras. This type of yoga practice includes both asanas and pranayama.

Anusara: The founder of this style of hatha yoga is the American, John Friend, a student of famous yoga guru B.K.S. Iyengar. This style of yoga is anatomically-based. In this style, emphasis is given on opening the heart. This style requires extensive teacher training. In the Anusara class of yoga, movements are coordinated with breath.

Ashtanga: The founder of this style of hatha yoga is K. Pattabhi Jois, a student of Sri T. Krishmanacharya. This style of yoga depends on specific sequence and continuous movement. It is very strenuous. This style of yoga is a combination of dynamic breathing and movement, heating the body in order to purify the blood, organs and nervous system and thus creates transformation from the inside out.

There are six series of Ashtang yoga. Generally, primary series (1st three) are practiced by beginners and the intermediate (4th series) and advanced series (5th and sixth series) should be practiced by perfectionists.

Bikram/Hot: The founder of this style of hatha yoga is Bikram Choudhury. This style of yoga consists of twenty-six postures and two breathing techniques. It is conducted for ninety minutes, in a room heated to 105°F (40.6°C), with a humidity of 40% to expel toxins and increase mobility.

Integral: The founder of this style of hatha yoga is Swami Satchidananda, a student of Swami Sivananda. This style of yoga includes gentle practice including postures, breathing, chants, and meditation.

Iyengar: The founder of this style of hatha yoga is B.K.S. Iyengar, a student of Sri T. Krishmanacharya. This style of yoga is based on strong anatomical basis and uses props to individualize postures. In this style of yoga, poses are held much longer than in other styles of yoga, in an effort to pay closer attention to the precise musculoskeletal alignment within each asana.

Kripalu: The founder of this style of hatha yoga is Amrit Desai, a student of Sri Kripalvananda. This style of yoga is taught in three stages with evolving emphasis. Stage one is focused on learning postures and understanding the body. This style of yoga develops a consciousness about the way you think, act, and feel not only in your practice, but in your day-to-day life as well.

Kundalini: The founder of this style of hatha yoga is Yogi Bhajan. This style of yoga is intended to awaken latent spiritual energy through postures, breathing and meditation.

This style of yoga builds physical vitality and increase consciousness.

Sivananda: The founder of this style of hatha yoga is Swami Vishnudevananda, a student of Swami Sivananda. This style of yoga contains gentle practice including twelve asanas, breathing, chants, and meditation. This style of yoga strengthen bones and boosts the circulatory and immune systems.

The twelve asanas include:

1. Sirshasana
2. Sarvangasana
3. Halasana
4. Matsyasana
5. Paschimothanasana
6. Bhujangasana
7. Shalabhasana
8. Dhanurasana
9. Ardh matsyendrasana
10. Padhastasana
11. Trikonasana
12. Shavasana

With regular practice one can ensure overall physical and mental health and the possible prevention of diseases such as diabetes, hypertension and arthritis.

2. Raja Yoga: This yoga is practiced by people who are using meditation for a higher achievement than only physical and mental fitness. This type of yoga is used by people who have a religious bent of mind and want to immerse themselves in long and deep meditation. This is a branch of yoga that is practiced by sages.

3. Jnana Yoga: Jnana means wisdom in Sanskrit language and hence this type of yoga concentrates on learning. Jnana yoga is one of the most difficult of the yoga practices as this involves the study of the ancient scriptures besides practicing yoga physically. This type of yoga concentrates on the development of the intellect of an individual and his/her connection with the larger universe as a whole.

4. Karma Yoga: If you can joyfully involve yourself in any activity that is karma yoga. If you do it with great effort, only karma will come, no yoga will happen. This is another branch of yoga which is mostly practiced by those who renounced the worldly life and want to lead an ascetic life. Karma yoga promotes selfless service and care for the less fortunate as devotion to God.

5. Bhakti Yoga: Bhakti means 'devotion' and hence this branch of yoga is dedicated to the love of God and through it, love of all life and mankind. This is a form of meditation which concentrates on channelizing all the energy towards becoming more loving and tolerant of others.

6. Mantra Yoga: Mantra yoga is a type of yoga that uses mantras to awaken the self and deepen the meditative aspects of a physical yoga practice. Mantra yoga is an exact science that is meant to engage the mind through focusing on sound, duration and number of repetitions. Repetition of the mantras is a means to get closer to the divinity within, and it creates positive vibrations that benefit both the one who chants and the one who listens.

No matter what type of yoga you choose, you would need to practice it daily and very seriously. If practiced correctly, yoga could get you rid of the majority of common ailments and keep you fit enough both mentally and physically to achieve the best results in anything you do in your life.

References

1. Gass R. Chanting: Discovering Spirit in Sound. New York NY: Broadway Books, 1999.
2. Campbell D. The Mozart Effect: Tapping the power of music to heal the body, strengthen the mind, and unlock the creative spirit. New York, NY: Avon Books, 1997.
3. White G. Yoga beyond belief: Insights to awaken and deepen your practice. North Atlantic Books; 2007.
4. Stephens M. Teaching yoga: Essential foundations and techniques. North Atlantic Books; 2011 Sep 6.

5. Iyengar BK. Light on yoga: yoga dīpikā. Schocken Books; 1970.
6. Iyengar BK. BKS Iyengar yoga: The path to holistic health. Penguin; 2007 Dec 17.

2
Physiological basis of Asana and Pranayama

Yoga is the most ancient Indian system for physical, mental and spiritual well-being in the world. The Sanskrit meaning of the word is union of the individual self with the Supreme Self. The different systems of yoga have techniques and practices ranging from physical postures (asanas), to the deepest stages of meditation, all aimed toward helping a person achieve optimum physical, mental and spiritual wellbeing.

Physiological basis of Yogasana

According to Patanjali's Yoga darshan, an asana is defined as **"Sthira sukham asanam"** which means any posture that can be maintained with comfort is an asana.

Yogasana can be divided into two categories

1. Which requires a sustained muscle contraction. For example, Trikonasan, Matsyasana, Salabhasana and Dhanurasana. These asanas are anaerobic exercises.

Yoga asana helps musculoskeletal system in many ways such as muscles, tendons and ligaments act on the bones to give the body its shape and posture. Yoga asanas can help redress problems associated with poor body posture and the effects of structural decay, because they strengthen weak muscles and stretch tight ones.

2. The second type of Asanas does not require any sustained muscular effort. Such asanas are good for meditation and *aum* chanting. Yoga-asanas help by keeping the body flexible, strong and balanced,

not only healthier but it also helps the yoga meditation practitioner to sit (or stand) comfortably when meditating.

Asanas

Asanas done lying supine

Naukasana: Naukasana strengthen the psoas major muscle. This muscle lies inside the abdomen and is not visible from outside.

Pawan muktasana: It improves flexibility of the spine.

Sarvangasana: Sarvangasana has more visceral than musculoskeletal effects. For example it facilitates drainage of secretions in the trachea-bronchial tree, in case of impaired muco-ciliary elevator. This asana is beneficial for the GI tract as it facilitates the movement of air bubbles in the stomach to the pyloric region inhibiting thereby the infectious organisms such as *Helicobactor pylori*. It causes peptic ulcers and in longer run gastric cancer. Air move down the duodenum to the colon thereby inhibiting anaerobic bacteria including *Entamoeba histolytica*. The air is ultimately passed down as flatus.

Halasana: Halasana stretches the dorsal spinal ligaments and improves spinal flexibility.

Asanas done in sitting posture

Paschimottanasana: It increases flexibility of the spine by putting stress on the posterior spinal ligaments.

Padmasana: It is a posture for practising concentration, which leads to parasympathetic activation.

Vajrasana: It keeps anaerobic load on the quadriceps muscles: Those fibers of the quadriceps muscle which contract in the almost fully flexed position of the knee, become stronger.

Ustrasana: This asana strengthens the metatarsal bones.

Matsyasana: It improves flexibility of the cervical spine. It stretches the oesophagus.

Asanas done lying prone

Bhujangasana: It improves the backward flexibility of the spine. Bhujangasana also stretches the oesophagus.

Shalabahasana: It increases the venous return to the heart.

Dhanurasana: It stretches the anterior spinal ligaments and also stretches the oesophagus and may be useful in conditions like hiatus hernia.

Asanas done in standing posture

Tadasana: It strengthens the small bones of the feet, metatarsals.

Vrkshasana: Improves balancing skill and strengthen the muscles of lower limbs.

Trikonasana: It builds up the anaerobic capacity of the quadriceps muscles and make them stronger.

Advanced Asanas

Chakrasana: It puts anaerobic load on and builds up the extensor muscles of the arm, muscle around shoulder, the quadriceps femoris, the glutei and the paraspinal muscles.

Mayurasana: It strengthens the fore arm muscles. In this asana, radius and ulna bear the whole body weight and are thus strengthened.

Sirsasana: It puts the whole body's weight on the cervical vertebrae and thus strengthens them. The circulatory, respiratory and gastrointestinal systems are benefited with this asana.

Asanas for relaxation

Makarasana: It helps in regulating the GI tract system.

Savasana: In this asana actively and deliberately relaxing each and every muscle of the body reduces the proprioceptive input to the central nervous system, thus gradually bringing down the sympathetic vasoconstrictior tone and reducing the resting blood pressure.

Physiological benefits of Pranayama

Regular practising of Pranayama can regulate vital gases such as oxygen and carbon dioxide. Pranayama, a type of yogic breathing may cause the changes in pressure of chest cavity where heart and lungs are positioned. The blood availability to hearts may be changed due to pressure variation in chest cavity, and therefore, breathing influences the heart which may lead to change in blood circulation and ultimately may affect the brain. Pranayama has capacity to influence and improve the vital parameters of the heart and lung.

Inhalation leads to increased heart rate while exhalation slows down the heart rate in every respiratory cycle. This coupling of inhale, exhale and heart rate is under the autonomic control. As a person becomes older, this coupling of inhale, exhale and heart rate decreases. Though, respiration is an automatic act, however one may have a great degree of voluntary control by practicing pranayama.

The slow breathing pranayama such as anulom-vilom is most beneficial in lowering hypertension. It reduces heart rate and blood pressure in patients of hypertension. Pranayama also has positive effects on brain. It influences the alertness, cognition, memory and behaviour. There are several studies which suggest that Pranayama can alleviate anxiety, depression and stress.

Therefore Pranayama or yogic breathing has capability to influence physiological systems. It may be useful in different types of diseases.

Pranayama leads to slower and deeper breathing: An expert in pranayama, compared to other people, tend to take fewer breaths of greater volume according to a study published in 1998 in *the Lancet*, performed on people with breathing problems due to congestive heart failure (CHF). In advanced CH, fluid can accumulate in the lungs interfering with normal oxygenation, creating a feeling of suffocation. The natural response is to get agitated and breathe very quickly to try to get in as much air as possible, but it turns out that this is counterproductive. Many rapid, shallow breaths actually deliver less air to the alveoli, the tiny air sacs in the lungs where oxygen exchange happens, than a few slower, deeper breaths. After one month of practicing a pranayama, patients in the study dropped from an average of 13.4 breaths/minute to 7.6. While their exercise capacity increased significantly, as did the oxygen saturation of their blood. Indeed, patients who started out feeling so short of breath that they were breathing more than twenty times per minute wound up with higher levels of oxygen in their blood by taking only six yogic breaths per minute.

Pranayama encourages breathing through nose: Regular practicing of yoga promotes breathing through the nose on both inhalation and exhalation. The nasal passages filter, warm, and humidify the air, removing some of the pollutants one may inhaled before they get to the lungs. Warm and moist air is less likely to set off an asthma attack. Nasal passages are narrower than the mouth, there is more resistance to air flow in them, which tends to slow the breath, calming the nervous system and the brain.

In conclusion, slow type pranayama improves cardiovascular health and autonomic conditioning, while fast breathing pranayama such as kapalbhati provides benefits for central nervous system.

References

1. McCall, Timothy. *Yoga as Medicine: The Yogic Prescription for Health and Healing.* New York: Bantam, 2007.
2. Prakash C Malshe. A medical understanding of Yoga. Antar prakashan centre for yoga. 2012.
3. Payne, Larry, et al. *Yoga Therapy and Integrative Medicine: Where Ancient Science Meets Modern Medicine.* Nashville, TN: Basic Health Publications, Inc., 2015.

❐

3
Yoga, Meditation and Mind-Body Health

Meditation is a practice where an individual trains his/her mind or induces a mode of consciousness, either to realize some benefit or for the mind to simply acknowledge its content without becoming identified with that content, or as an end in itself. Meditation can be done right before or after a physical yoga practice. Sit with good posture either on the floor, cross-legged, or in a chair if it's more comfortable. Meditation practice improves a wide range of willpower skills, including alertness, focus, stress management, impulse control and self-awareness. It changes both the function and structure of the brain to support self-control. For example, regular meditators have more gray matter in the prefrontal cortex. Several studies suggest that meditation is about way more than blissing out.

Mechanism of Mind-Body Communication

Nerve cells in the brain thought and feeling centers connect to other nerve cells in the brain and body, Hormone - producing tissues and organs, and immune cells throughout the body. In this way, mental activity is able to influence many of the body's physiological processes and thereby affect health.

The brain automatically regulates essential functions of the body such as breathing, digestion, blood pressure and blood flow, and reaction to the environment. Most brain activities occur without conscious control. But the mind can be trained through various mental and physical techniques to be more effective in healing illnesses and injuries. On the other hand, if your mind is disturbed, anxious, or depressed, it can cause bodily organs to malfunction. In other way, human mind can cause changes in body chemistry through thoughts and feelings, which may have a positive or negative effect on your health.

A key to maintaining or improving health and wellness is to learn and practice a mental relaxation technique such as meditation.

- Meditation does not have to be done in religious settings, nor is it complicated.
- For meditating choose a quiet place in your home or outside.
- Sit in a comfortable position with your back straight.
- Be sure that you have at least 10 to 30 minutes during which you will not be disturbed.
- If you are busy and not finding time, then you can meditate before bedtime.

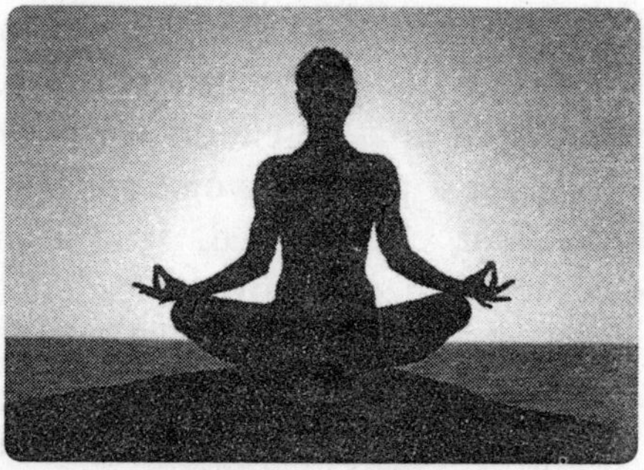

What are the Benefits of Meditation?

Meditation may lead to the sense of calm, peace and balance that can benefit physical and emotional well-being. The benefits are not only limited to when your meditation session ends. Meditation can help you carry on more calmly through your day and may help you manage symptoms of certain medical conditions.

Meditation and Emotional Well-being

When you meditate, you may clear away the information overload that builds up every day and contributes to your stress. The emotional benefits of meditation can include:

- Gaining a new perspective on stressful situations
- Building skills to manage your stress
- Increasing self-awareness
- Focusing on the present

- Reducing negative emotions
- Increasing imagination and creativity
- Increasing patience and tolerance

What will be the Effect of meditation on Illness?

Stress related problems may be curtailed by meditation. A large number of researchers support that meditation improves stress related problems while, some researchers believe it is not yet possible to draw conclusions about the possible benefits of meditation.

Some researchers suggest that meditation may help people manage symptoms of conditions such as anxiety, asthma, cancer, chronic pain, depression, heart disease, high blood pressure, irritable bowel syndrome, sleep problems and headaches due to tension. Meditation is not a replacement for traditional medical treatment. But it may be a useful addition to your other treatment.

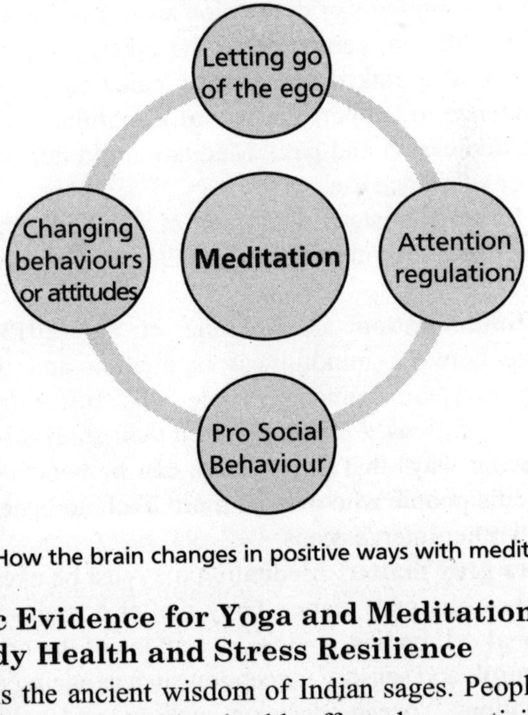

Fig: How the brain changes in positive ways with meditation!

Scientific Evidence for Yoga and Meditation Improve Mind-body Health and Stress Resilience

Yoga is the ancient wisdom of Indian sages. People experience energetic, fresh and positive health effects by practicing yoga and meditation. Practicing Yoga leads to both mental and physical benefits. However, we still hav e much to learn about how exactly these practices affect mind-body health. A new research article published in Frontiers in Human Neuroscience investigates the effects of yoga and meditation on brain derived neurotrophic factor (BDNF), the activity on the hypothalamic pituitary adrenal (HPA) effects and inflammatory markers. By studying the participants of an intensive 3-month yoga and meditation retreat, the researchers found that the yoga practices positively impacted BDNF signaling, the cortisol awakening response and immunological markers, and in addition improved subjective wellbeing.

In a meta-analyses, Goyel et.al (2013) reported that mindfulness meditation may be useful in battles against anxiety, depression and pain. Using data from 47 earlier studies, Goyal and his team found between a 5 and 10 percent improvement in anxiety symptoms among people who took part in mindfulness meditation, compared to those who did another activity. There was also about a 10 to 20 percent improvement in symptoms of depression among those who practiced mindfulness meditation, compared to the other group. Mindfulness meditation was also linked to reduced pain. Goyel et al. found moderate evidence to support the use of mindfulness meditation to treat anxiety, depression and pain. Meditation did not seem to affect mood, sleep or substance use.

Boosts immune system: Davidson et al. (2003) showed a link between an eight-week mindfulness meditation program and better immune function.

Eases inflammation: Rosenkranz et al. (2013) identified a possible tie between mindfulness meditation and the relief of inflammatory symptoms among people who suffer from chronic inflammatory conditions. Authors reported their study does show that there are specific ways that mindfulness can be beneficial, and that there are specific people who may be more likely to benefit from this approach than other interventions.

Increases gray matter: Meditation may just be exercise for the brain to increase the gray matter. Grey matter contains most of the brain's neuronal cell bodies. It includes regions of the brain involved in muscle control, and sensory perception such as seeing and hearing, memory, emotions, speech, decision making, and self-control. In a study Kurth et al. (2014) showed that MRI scans of long-time meditators revealed that certain parts of their brains were larger than those of a control group, particularly in regions known for emotion regulation. Another small study published in 2011 in the journal Psychiatry Research by Holzel et al (2011) reported that neuroimaging showed that an eight-week mindfulness-based stress reduction program resulted in increases in gray matter in the hippocampus and areas of the brain tied to compassion and self-awareness.

Builds Self-knowledge: According to Carlson (2013), mindfulness (defined as "paying attention to one's current experience in a non-judgmental way") can help people to understand their own personalities. For example, one who overestimates the positivity of his or her personality or status is often disliked by others, whereas having insight into how others perceive the self and acknowledging one's flaws seems to attenuate the negativity of others' impressions.

Builds focus and concentration: A study by Mac Lean et al. (2010) reported that Buddhist meditation improved focus and attention on a task that was designed to be both boring and demanding. "People may think meditation is something that makes you feel good and going on a meditation retreat is like going on vacation, and you get to be at peace with yourself."

Boosts cognitive function: Mrazek et al. (2013) in their study identified a link between mindfulness training and increased standardized test scores, as well as improvements in working memory. Authors reported that regular meditation may stave off the thinning of the brain's prefrontal cortex, and in turn declines in cognitive function, later in life.

Helps in getting better sleep: Meditation may be an effective behavioral intervention in the treatment of insomnia, according to a research abstract presented on June 9, at Sleep 2009, the 23rd Annual Meeting of the Associated Professional Sleep Societies.

In summary, you become more aware of the power your mind has to improve health, healing and help you perform better and help prevent sickness. Practicing daily meditation in a quiet place will improve mind and body harmony which will release good chemicals in the body and you will feel better and perform well in your all tasks.

References

1. B. Rael Cahn, Matthew S. Goodman, Christine T. Peterson, Raj Maturi, Paul J. Mills. Yoga, Meditation and Mind-Body

Health: Increased BDNF, Cortisol Awakening Response, and Altered Inflammatory Marker Expression after a 3-Month Yoga and Meditation Retreat. Frontiers in Human Neuroscience, 2017; 11 DOI: 10.3389/fnhum.2017.00315.

2. Madhav Goyal, Sonal Singh, Erica M. S. Sibinga, Neda F. Gould, Anastasia Rowland-Seymour, Ritu Sharma, Zackary Berger, Dana Sleicher, David D. Maron, Hasan M. Shihab, Padmini D Ranasinghe, Shauna Linn, Shonali Saha, Eric B. Bass, Jennifer A. Haythornthwaite. Meditation Programs for Psychological Stress and Well-being: A Systematic Review and Meta-analysis. JAMA Intern Med. 2014 Mar; 174(3): 357–368.
3. Davidson RJ, Kabat-Zinn J, Schumacher J, Rosenkranz M, Muller D, Santorelli SF, Urbanowski F, Harrington A, Bonus K, Sheridan JF. Alterations in brain and immune function produced by mindfulness meditation. Psychosom Med. 2003 Jul-Aug; 65(4):564-70.
4. Rosenkranz MA, Davidson RJ, Maccoon DG, Sheridan JF, Kalin NH, Lutz A. A comparison of mindfulness-based stress reduction and an active control in modulation of neurogenic inflammation. Brain Behav Immun. 2013 Jan;27(1):174-84.
5. Kurth F, Luders E, Wu B, Black DS. Brain Gray Matter Changes Associated with Mindfulness Meditation in Older Adults: An Exploratory Pilot Study using Voxel-based Morphometry. Neuro. 2014;1(1):23-26.
6. Holzel BK1, Carmody J, Vangel M, Congleton C, Yerramsetti SM, Gard T, Lazar SW. Mindfulness practice leads to increases in regional brain gray matter density. Psychiatry Res. 2011 Jan 30;191(1):36-43.
7. Carlson EN. Overcoming the Barriers to Self-Knowledge: Mindfulness as a Path to Seeing Yourself as You Really Are. Perspectives on Psychological Science, 2013; 8 (2): 173
8. Mac Lean KA, Ferrer E, Aichele SR, Bridwell DA, Zanesco AP, Jacobs TL, King BG,Rosenberg EL, Sahdra BK, Shaver PR, Wallace BA, Mangun GR, Saron CD. Intensive meditation training improves perceptual discrimination and sustained attention. Psychol Sci. 2010 Jun;21(6):829-39.

9. Mrazek MD, Franklin MS, Phillips DT, Baird B, Schooler JW. Mindfulness training improves working memory capacity and GRE performance while reducing mind wandering. Psychol Sci. 2013 May;24(5):776-81.
10. Gordon Edin and Eric Golanty. Health and wellness. 12th Edition, Jones & Bartlett Learning, 2015

❐

4
Stress Management through Yoga

Stress may be defined as the sum of physical and emotional reactions to any stimulus that disturbs the harmony of mind and body. The body's response towards stress can be influenced by one's experiences, genetics, and behavior. When the brain perceives stress, physiological and behavioral responses are initiated leading to the adaptation. (Fig. 1). Stressful thoughts trigger the release of a hormone called

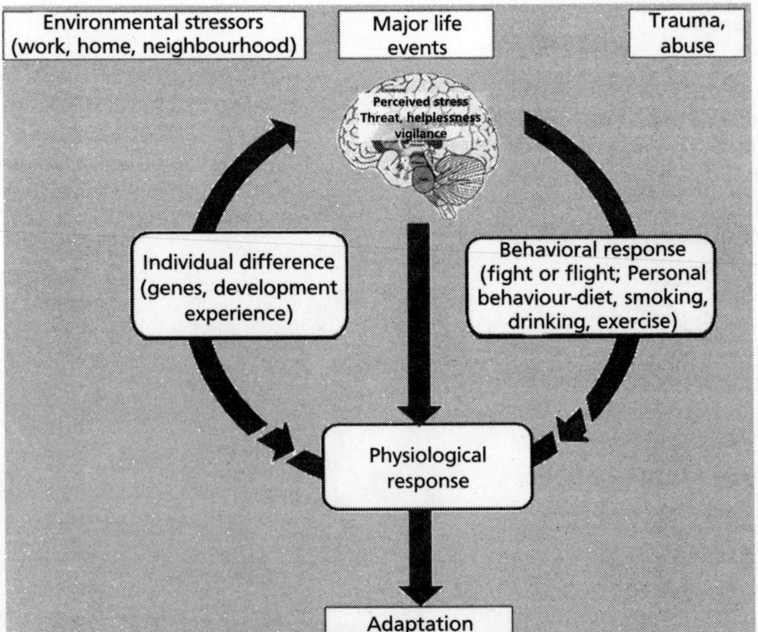

Fig. 1: Stress Response

corticotrophin releasing factor (CRF) from the hypothalamus of the brain. CRF flows in the blood stream to the pituitary gland, where it stimulates the release of cortisol and other stress hormones. In acute stress, cortisol helps prepare the body for fight, flight, wound healing, and infection. In chronic stress, cortisol unbalances metabolism and suppresses the immune system. However, acute stress causes immune enhancing effects by causing lymphocyte and macrophage redistribution throughout the body. This trafficking is mediated by glucocorticoids. The immune enhancing effects of acute stress depend on adrenal secretion and last for three to five days. In a nut shell, acute stress could be immune stimulatory while chronic stress leads to suppressed immunity.

How does Stress Occurs?

Stress results from the interplay of stressful environmental situation and the mental, emotional and physiological reactions to those occurrences (Fig. 2).

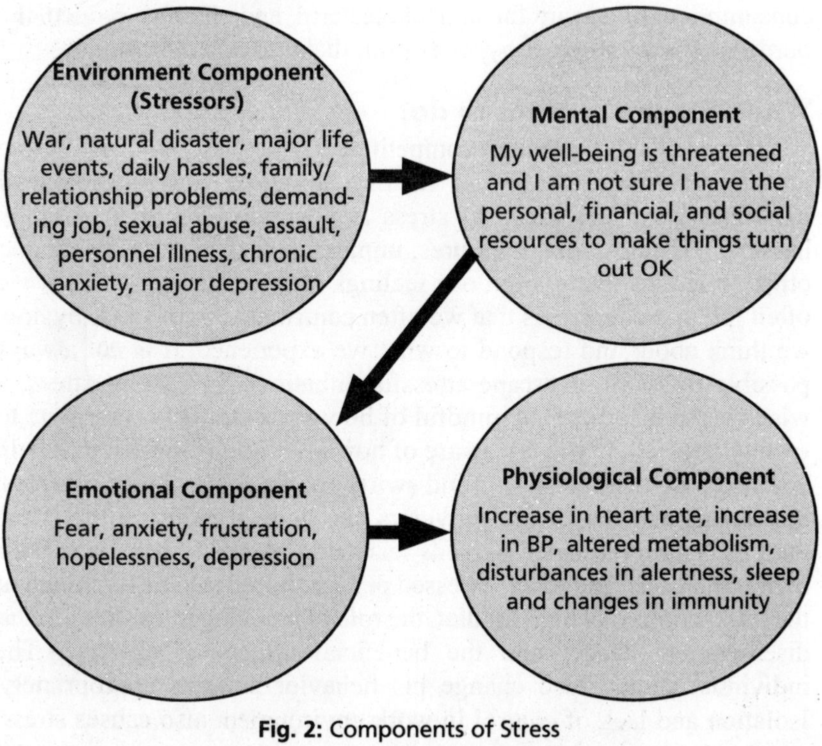

Fig. 2: Components of Stress

How does Stress Contribute to Illness from Wellness?

Chronic stress may lead to illness by (1) causing the mind and body to become exhausted, (2) weakening immunity and (3) motivating unhealthy behaviours in an attempt to deal with stress. Several studies have shown that stress can impair the person's immunity. For example, students who experience considerable stress prior to taking exams show reduced blood levels of natural killer (NK) cells, and T cells thus stress generated due to exam makes susceptible to the colds and flu. Stress related impairment of the immune system is mediated by cortisol, one of the stress hormones which bind to immune cells and alter their functions. Overall, chronic stress weakens your immunity which leads to the chronic illness. Chronic diseases are the leading cause of death throughout the world. It reduces the quality of life of the affected person for many years. Chronic diseases are also associated with five risk factors: tobacco use, high blood pressure, alcohol use, high cholesterol and overweight. To reduce the burden of chronic diseases, individuals must be encouraged and taught how to be healthier and restrict the use of tobacco and alcohol. Limit the consumption of sugar, fat and cholesterol and thereby reduce the burdens of heart disease, hypertension, diabetes and overweight.

When Stressed, what to do?

In today's fast growing, competitive world it is almost impossible not to experience stress and its psychological and physiological manifestations. The cause of stress is generally identified as daily hassles, obstacles, time pressures, unpleasantness in relationship and other situations that disrupt our feelings of inner harmony. What we often fail to recognize, is that we often contribute to our stress by how we think about and respond to what we experience. It is not always possible to avoid or escape stressful situations. In case of stress, a wise course is to become mindful of how your thoughts contribute to feeling stressed. If you are aware of how your mind works it will help you decrease the time your mind swirls around in the throes of stress. Physicians and healthcare providers can help in reducing the stress load by helping affected persons learn coping skills, recognize their own limitations, and relax. Stressed person should also be reminded of the interactions of a high fat diet, the role of smoking in cardiovascular diseases and cancer and the beneficial effects of exercise. The individual should also change his behavior patterns appropriately. Isolation and lack of control in work environment also causes stress.

Interventions that increase social support and enhance coping prolong illnesses also improved the health and attitude towards work and one such intervention is yoga.

Stress Management by Yoga

In yoga, breathing can stimulate the vagus nerve and help reduce stress. Vagus nerve is the main nerve of parasympathetic nervous system, extends from medulla through the diaphragm to abdomen and responsible for (i) slowing respiration (ii) reducing heart rate (iii) lowering blood pressure and (iv) stimulating digestive activity. Yoga for stress management is successful because of the balance created in the nervous and endocrine systems — directly influence all the other systems and organs of the body. Yoga has been considered as universal remedy for stress. In this context, we will discuss the role of yoga in developing a healthy lifestyle by which stress can be managed. Yoga can play an important role in stress management.

Yoga is not limited to the physical postures, breathing techniques or meditation only, rather yoga is a way of life also. It propounds several principles including asana, pranayama, kriya, mudra, bandha and meditation which are relevant to healthy living. Yogic principles of healthy living can be adopted by all, irrespective of age, gender, profession or place.

As a way of life, yoga gives direction about food, eating habits, thinking, recreational means and conduct. Yogic way of life, if adopted in the true sense, empowers us to deal with stress and in promoting physical and mental health. The components of yogic way of life are:

- Ahara (Food)
- Vihara (Relaxation)
- Achara (Conduct)
- Vichara (Thinking)
- Vyavahara (Behaviour or actions)

Ahara (Food)

The principles of *ahara* are related to food consumption. Yoga emphasises on *mitahara*, which are related to quality and quantity of food and also the state of mind during the intake of food. Proper diet is an integral part of yoga. Food is the substance that keeps the body healthy and alive, but it can also be the source of substances that may be harmful for the body.

Food serves several purposes in our lives. It provides energy to perform our daily chores, helps build resistance to infections and even makes us happy.

The type of food you eat determines the type of mind you have. As the food, so the mind; as the mind, so the man. Eat easily digestible food i.e. Sattvic food which includes: Milk and milk products, fresh fruits and dry fruits, seasonal vegetables, cereals such as wheat, unpolished rice, jowar, bajra, corn, Pulses - moong dal - green with skin and yellow, sprouted cereals and pulses, a little ginger, turmeric powder (haldi), cumin seeds (jeera), coriander powder (dhania). Honey, jaggery, crystal sugar (misry), raw sugar (shud shakkar) ghee or rice bran oil, filtered oil - (groundnut or till oil). Eating this kind of simple food brings relaxation and a feeling of peace. Mitahar emphasises the right quantity and quality of food eaten in positive state of mind.

Vihara (Relaxation)

The English meaning of Vihara is relaxation which can be brought by activities such as exercise, recreation and some creative activities like drawing, painting, singing, etc. These activities not only help us to regulate and channelize our emotions but also are a source of joy and happiness in our life. Doing yogic practices such as practice of asanas, pranayama and meditation help in relaxing our body and our mind, also relaxation can be attained in a good company as well. Sound sleep is also an important thing for relaxation. It is, therefore important that we should regularly follow a timetable that provides an adequate time for yogic as well as creative activities.

Achara (Conduct)

Achara with meaning as right conduct including emotions, attitudes, desires, instincts, and habits is essential for a stress free life. The positivity of emotions and attitudes, good habits and controlling our desires helps to make us strong not only individually but also socially; also we get protected from the unnecessary stress by the right Achara. That is why one should have control on one's desires, instincts, emotions, habits and attitudes. Yoga, having the property to have a good conduct in one's personal and social life is very important to us, also Yoga advocates positivity of emotions and attitudes towards self and also towards others. The principles of Yoga that are helping us in developing a control on our desires as well as emotions and bringing peace and harmony are YAMA (restraint) and NIYAMA (observance).

Vichara (Thoughts)

As we know that there is a huge importance of thoughts in our life as they act like a guide to our behaviour, which means the behaviour of a human depends upon the thoughts he is having. So one should always think positive. As we know there are two sides of each similarly, positive thoughts are able to bring happiness in our life while negative thoughts can be a source of unhappiness in our life. The right thinking has many advantages like, it provides appropriate behaviour to a human, it prevents and manages stress related health problems. In Yoga, it is prescribed that one should have positivity in their thoughts as positive thoughts provide us the strength to overcome our sorrows of life. Doing yogic practices like Pratyahara and Dhyana (meditation) helps one in controlling thoughts and hence bringing optimism in life.

Vyavahara (Behaviour)

Vyavahara taking the meaning as actions is the result of Ahara, Vihara, Achara, Vichara. Yogic philosophy propounds that our actions should be right and should not be indulged in the wrong activities. One's behaviour towards others should be appropriate. One should perform right act with one's full dedication without worrying for the result of their actions as proposed by Karma Yoga one can remain stress free and be happy in his/her life if he/she follows the this philosophy act accordingly.

Asanas for Management of Stress

Some Asanas and Pranayam which are helpful in stress management are given below:

1. Hasta Utthanasana

Procedure

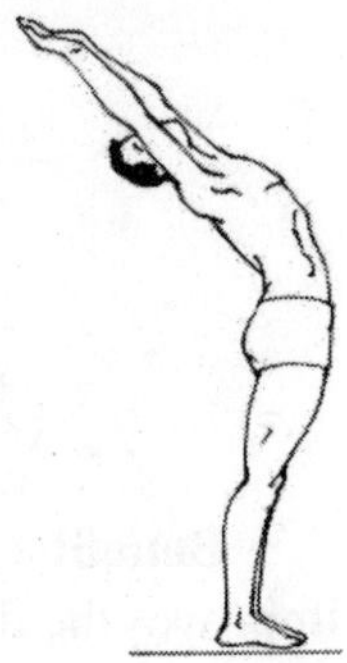

1. Separate the hands raise and stretch both arms above the head, keeping them shoulder width apart.
2. Bend the head, arms and upper trunk slightly backward.
3. Maintain this position comfortably for 5-10 seconds in the beginning.

Benefits: Improves digestion and lung capacity.

2. Padahastasana

Procedure

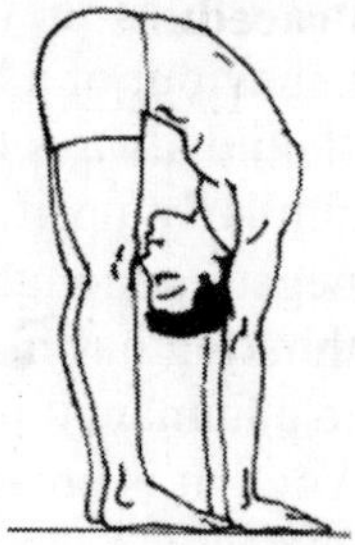

1. Bend forward from the hips until the fingers or palms of the hands touch the floor on either side of the feet.
2. Keep the knees straight and bring the forehead as close as possible to the knee.
3. Maintain this position comfortably for 10 to 15 seconds.

Benefits: Improves digestion, removes flatulence and indigestion. Increase flexibility of back and leg muscles.

3. Trikonasan

Procedure

1. Stand erect and keep distance between your legs about 3 to 4 feet.
2. Extend your arms at the shoulder level.
3. Inhale and raise your right arm by the side of your head.
4. Now, bend your right arms with exhaling towards the left side by keeping your body weight equally on both the feet. You should ensure that the right arm become parallel to the ground.
5. Maintain the position as per your comfort with normal breathing (for 5-10 seconds) and come to the original position by inhaling.
6. Do the same procedure with the left arm.

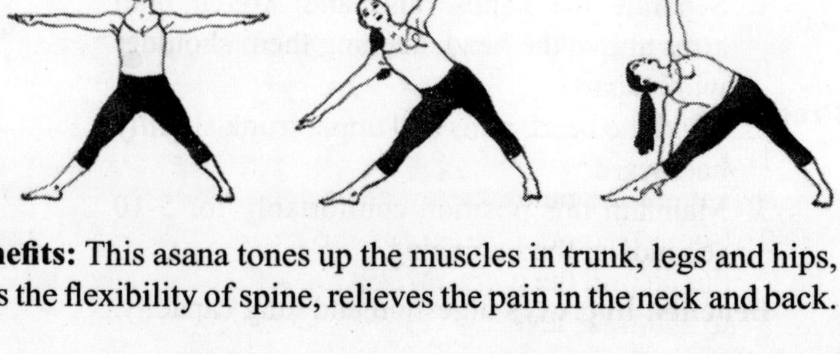

Benefits: This asana tones up the muscles in trunk, legs and hips, improves the flexibility of spine, relieves the pain in the neck and back.

4. Shashakasan

Procedure

1. Sit with your legs straight in front of you, keeping the palms near the buttocks.
2. Fold the right leg at the knee and place the foot below the right buttock – the sole should face outwards.
3. Similarly fold the left leg and place the foot below the left buttock with the sole facing outwards. The big toes should touch each other.
4. Raise both arms over the head.
5. Then keeping the arms straight, lower your body towards the floor. Rest your hands on the floor. Then try to touch either the forehead or the crown of the head on the floor. Ensure that your elbows are straight.
6. Close your eyes and maintain the pose for three to five breaths.
7. To come out of the asana, first lift your head off the floor, then raise the body and hands up. Slowly bring the hands down and rest them on the knees, come out of vajrasana and sit in a relaxed manner.

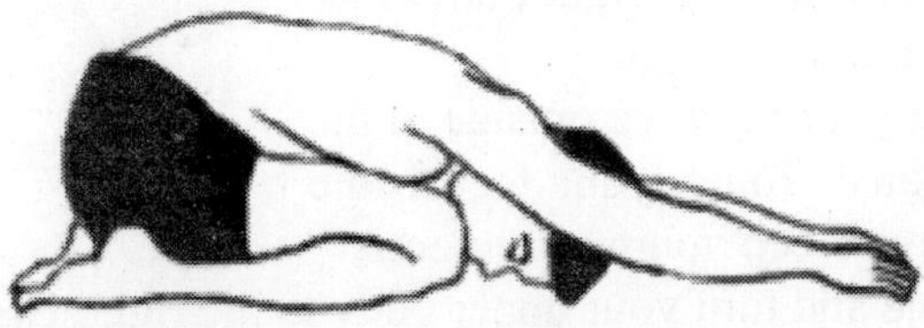

Benefits: It relaxes the body and helps in reducing the stress and improves the functioning of liver, kidneys and other visceral organs.

Note: Persons suffering from backache and cervical spondylitis should avoid this *asana*.

5. Ardha Ushtrasana (Half Camel Pose)

Procedure

1. Sit in vajrasana. Move the knees apart and the ankles to the side of the buttocks.
2. Stand up on the knees with the arms at the sides. Keep the feet flat behind the body. Stretch the arms sideways and raise them to shoulder level.

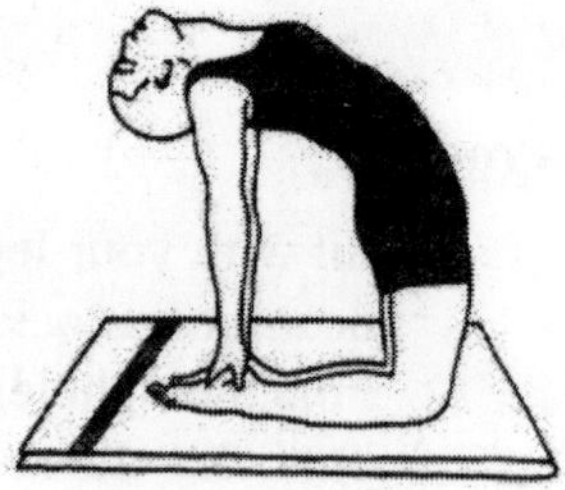

3. Twist to the right, reach back with the right hand and hold the right ankle.
4. Stretch the left arm, reach back and hold the left leg. The head should be slightly back with the eyes gazing at the upward. Push the hips forward in the final position and keep the thighs vertical.
5. Maintain the posture comfortably for 5-10 seconds.

Benefits: Improves the digestive system. Relieving backache and cures rounded back and drooping shoulders.

6. Ardhamatsyendrasana

Procedure

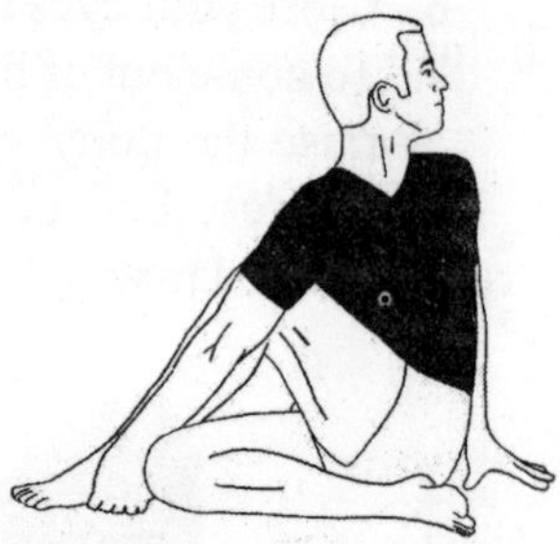

1. Sit in vajrasana position or sit straight with stretching your legs in front of you.
2. Bend your left leg and try to touch your feet to your right buttock as shown in the image.
3. Bring your right leg outside of the left knee. Touch your feet to the ground. Keep your spine erect.
4. Exhale and turn your upper body to the right. Hold your right feet with left hand and place your right hand behind you are on the ground as shown in the image.
5. Breathe normally and hold this posture for 20 to 30 seconds. After practicing you can hold this posture for 3 to 5 minutes.
6. Now release this posture and repeat this cycle with bending right leg and bringing left leg outside of the right knee. (i.e. Twisting the opposite direction).

Benefits: It relieves back pain, stimulates liver, spleen and pancreas and helps to regulate their functioning and benefits intestines also. It also strengthens the spinal column and muscles of the back.

7. Bhujangasan

Procedure

1. Lie down on abdomen with legs close together to the ground.
2. Place hands besides the body with palm touching on ground. Lift the prone body from the ground up to the naval region.
3. Maintain the position for 5-10 seconds or as long as comfortable.

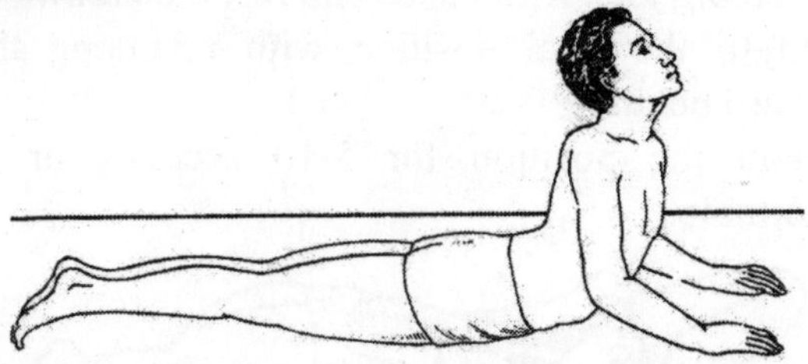

Benefits: Relieves constipation, indigestion and flatulence. Helps in improving lung function.

8. Makarasana (Crocodile pose)

Procedure

1. Lie down on abdomen with legs spread out, toes remain out and heels inward.
2. Slowly fold the left hand at below the armpit. Place it on the right shoulder.
3. Likewise place the right arm on the left shoulder.
4. Place the head on the hands in a comfortable position.
5. Maintain the position for 5-10 seconds or as long as comfortable.

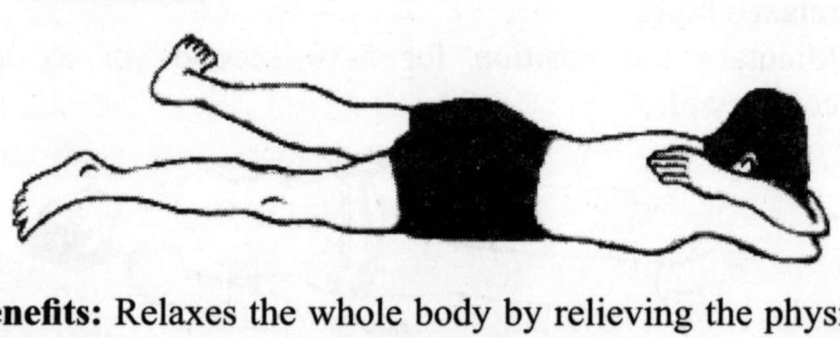

Benefits: Relaxes the whole body by relieving the physical and mental fatigue. It helps in relieving from back problems, helpful in coping with stress.

9. Matsyasana (Fish pose)

Procedure

1. Sit in Padmasana. Bend backward carefully supporting the body with the arms and elbows. With exhaling arch the back by lifting the neck and the chest, take the head back and rest the crown on the floor.
2. Hold the big toes with hands and rest the elbows on the floor.
3. Return to the final position with reversing the order of backward bending.
4. Maintain the position for 5-10 seconds or as long as comfortable.

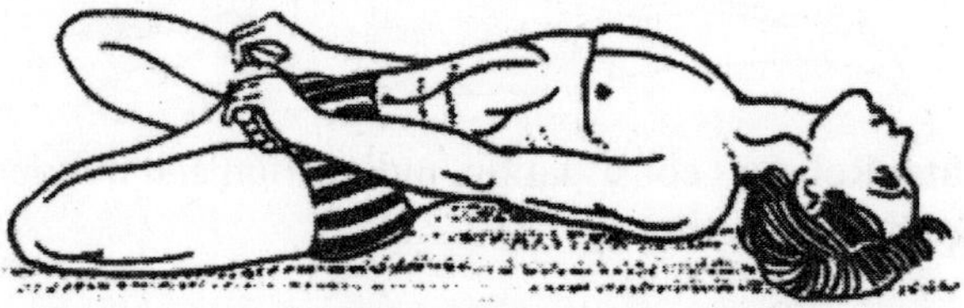

Benefits: Improves digestion and lung capacity. Increases flexibility of shoulder and back. Makes thyroid, parathyroid and adrenal gland healthy.

10. Shavasana (Corpse Pose)

Procedure

1. Lie down on back and place hands near the thighs and palm facing upwards.
2. Keep the heels slightly apart and toes pointing outwards with relaxed body.
3. Maintain the position for 5-10 seconds or as long as comfortable.

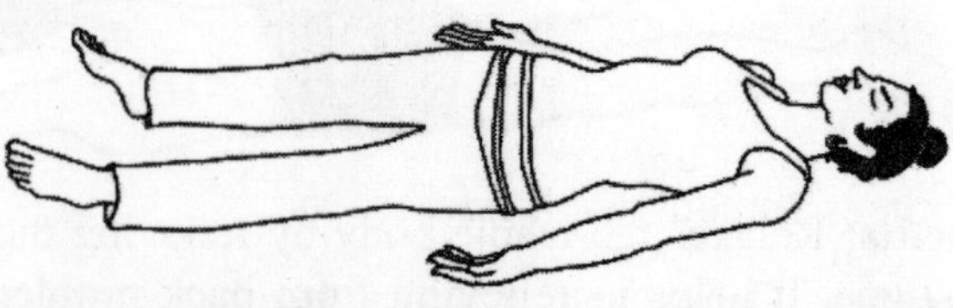

Benefits: Relaxes whole body. Relieves physical and mental fatigue. Extremely beneficial for high blood pressure and relieving stress.

Pranayama (Yoga Breathing Techniques)

Kapalbhati

Procedure

1. Sit in Padmasana, put both hands on respective knees. Exhale faster and forcibly through both the nostrils. Simultaneously draw the abdomen in.
2. After completing exhalation with force, take the breath in and bring the abdomen in previous position.
3. The sound produced during inhalation and exhalation should be like a bellows of the blacksmith.

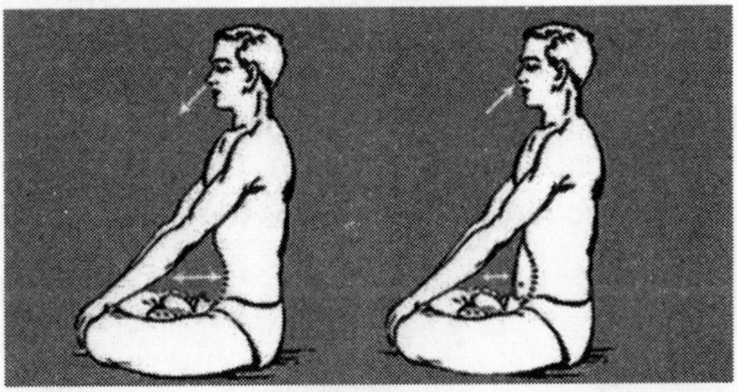

Benefits: Cleanses the naso-pharynx. Improves digestion.

Anulom-Viloma (Alternate Nostril Breathing)

Procedure

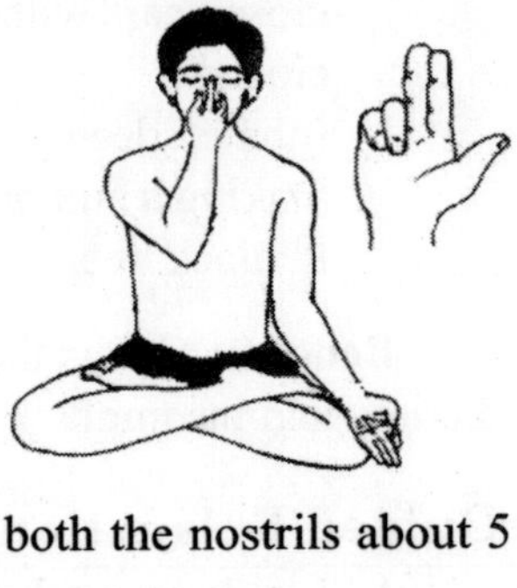

1. Sit in Padmasana with head and spine erect and eyes closed.
2. Close the right nostrils with the right thumb.
3. Inhale through the left nostril just before closing it with ring finger and release the air through the right nostril.
4. Repeat the process alternatively for both the nostrils about 5 times without making any sound.

Benefits: Calms and steadies the mind. Improves focus and concentration. Manages hypertension.

Bhastrika (bellows type breathing)

Procedure

1. Sit in a comfortable meditation posture with the hands resting on the knees.
2. Keep the head and spine straight, close the eyes and relax the whole body.
3. Take a deep breath in and breathe out forcefully through the nose.
4. Immediately afterwards, breath in with the same force. The force of inhalation and exhalation must be equal.
5. Continue in this manner, counting 10 breaths.
6. Take a deep breath in and breathe out slowly.

Benefits: This practice burns up toxins and helps balance the doshas or humours: kapha or phlegm, pitta or bile and vata or wind. Increases metabolic rate and improves digestion.

Bhramari

Procedure

1. Sit in the position of Padmasana.
2. Using both the hands, place index finger on the forehead, close eyes with middle finger and close years with thumbs with lips closed.
3. Inhale deeply and exhale by making a humming sound similar to black bee.

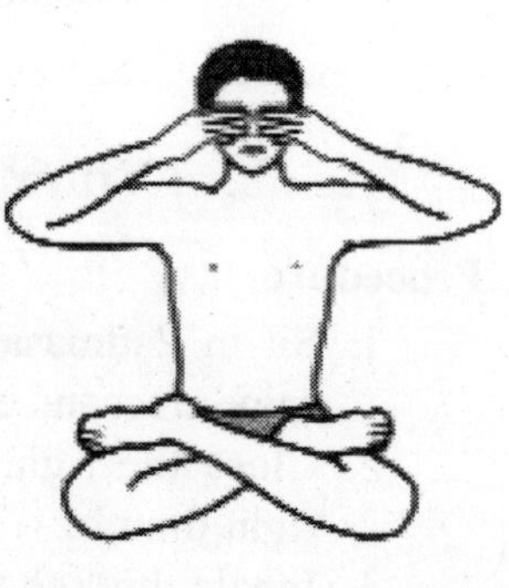

Benefits: Calms the mind and nervous system. Alleviates anger, anxiety and insomnia.

Guided Relaxation

1. Lie down on the ground. Keep a distance of one foot between the legs and keep both the hands open pointing upwards at some distance from the thighs.
2. Close the eyes, keep the neck straight and relax the whole body.

3. Gently inhale and exhale four to five deep breaths.
4. Now observe each part of the body through the mind with resolution and feeling that each part of the body is in a relaxed and stress-free state.
5. Do not sleep during the practice.

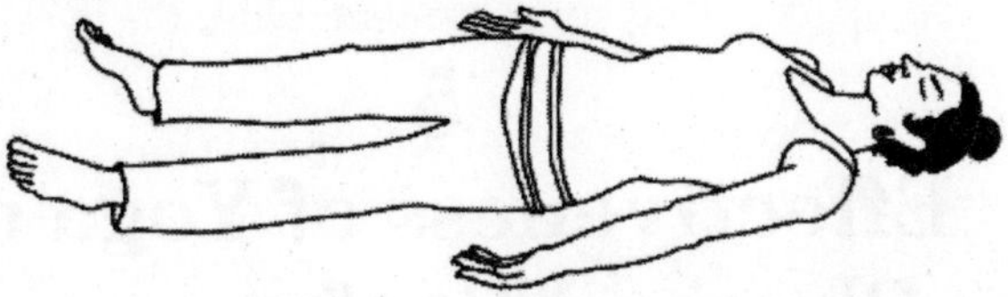

Benefits: Reduces mental stress, depression, high blood pressure, heart diseases and insomnia. The body, mind, brain and soul get complete rest, power, motivation and happiness. The concentration power is developed.

References

1. McCall, Timothy. *Yoga as Medicine: The Yogic Prescription for Health and Healing*. New York: Bantam, 2007.
2. Khalsa, Sat Bir, Cohen, Lorenzo, McCall, Timothy, Telles, Shirley. *The Principles and Practice of Yoga in Health Care.* Edinburgh: Handspring Publishing, 2016.
3. Payne, Larry, et al. *Yoga Therapy and Integrative Medicine: Where Ancient Science Meets Modern Medicine*. Nashville, TN: Basic Health Publications, Inc., 2015.

❒

5

Effectiveness of Yoga on Physical Performance and Well-being

Physical activity is anything you do when you are not sitting or lying down. Scientifically it is defined as "the amount of energy expended to produce movement". A movement occurs when energy derived from food is utilized by muscles that are connected to bones to shorten or lengthen. Physical activity is measured in terms of calories used per minute or metabolic equivalent or Physical activity level.

Calories used per minute: Physical activity can be measured in terms of calorie utilized in one minute for various physical activities.

Metabolic equivalent (MET): MET are per minute multiples of the amount of energy used while sitting or lying still, which is defines as 1MET.

Physical activity level: Physical activity level is the amount of daily energy expended over and above a person's basal or resting metabolism, which is the energy required to fuel basic life functions while at rest.

Yoga is a system of physical activity or exercise formulated in India thousands of years ago to unite one's mind and body. The principal physical benefits of yoga are enhancing muscular fitness and body flexibility. Yoga can help reduce risk factors for lifestyle diseases. Regular Yogic practices (Postures and Pranayam) facilitate better health, both as prevention and as treatment regimen that are supported by the scientific evidences.

There are many ways by which yoga served as preventive medicine for human well-being.

1. **Yogic practices increases flexibility:** Yoga and stretching goes hand in hand. The regular practicing of yogasanas can make body more flexible, giving a greater range of motion to the muscles and joints. A person having a flexible body is less prone to injuries because it can withstand physical stress. Lack of flexibility in the body may lead to several problems such as strain on knee joint; back pain etc.
2. **Muscle strengthening:** Strength training is a type of physical exercise specializing in the use of resistance to induce muscular contraction, which builds the strength, anaerobic endurance and size of skeletal muscles. This is exactly what your muscles are doing when you hold poses for extended periods of time. A study conducted by the University of Wisconsin's Human Performance Laboratory University, in which subjects practiced Hatha yoga for 55 minutes, three days a week for eight weeks, researchers noticed an improvement in their subjects' strength and endurance. Therefore, in addition to strengthening muscles, yoga appears to build endurance and delay the onset of fatigue.

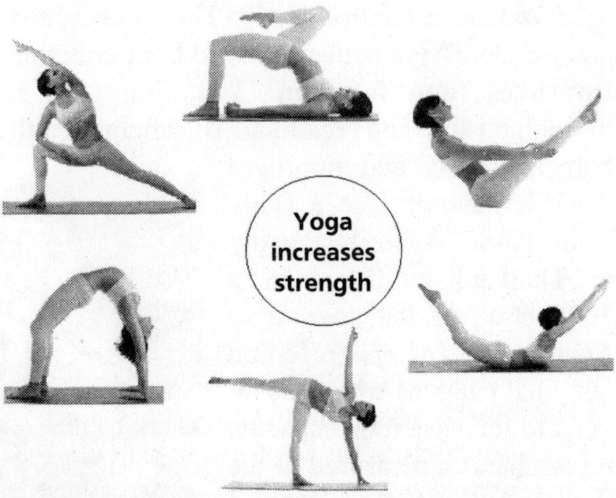

3. **Improves balance:** Yoga also help in balancing left to right and front to back, which can help minimize the muscle imbalance that so often leads to troublesome symptoms and injuries.

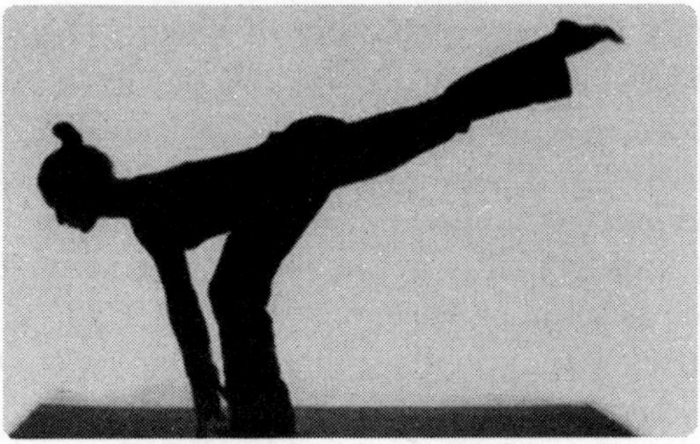

4. **Boosts immunity:** Scientific evidences supports that yoga improves immunity. A better immune system therefore prevents many a diseases which includes opportunistic infections, and diseases that occur by stressful environmental conditions. Meditation reported to be very effective in improving immunity as well as curtailing autoimmune diseases. A study conducted by University of Wisconsin examined a group of high tech workers who learned simple meditation technique and yoga postures, developed a higher level of influenza antibodies in their blood after getting a flu vaccine than a control group. This study showed that yoga practitioners have better ability to fight infection.
5. **Improves lung function:** Yoga improves lung function through posture and breathing. Yoga helps healthy people take bigger breaths and improves posture, according to a study from Khon Kaen University in Thailand published in a 2006 issue of the *Journal of Physiological Sciences*. To find out what happens when you do yoga to increase lung capacity, researchers measured the participant's chest expansion and lung volume rates at the beginning of the study and again six weeks later. The results showed the yoga group had significant improvement in lung volume and increased

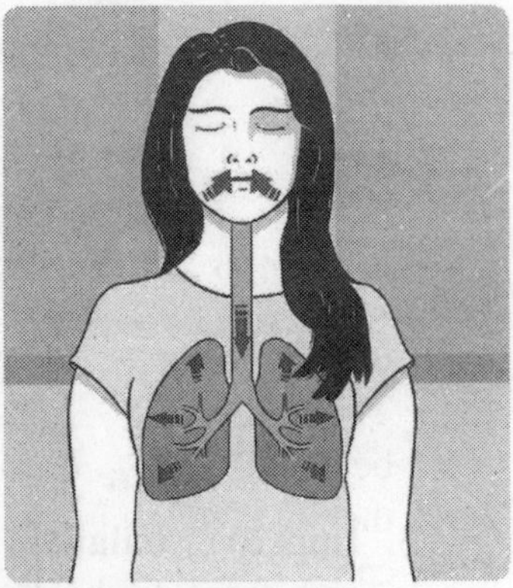

exhalation force, along with improved posture. Their chest wall expansion had increased 38 percent in the upper chest, 19 percent in the mid-chest and 15 percent in the lower chest.

6. **Increases oxygenation of tissues:** Yogic breathing supplies more oxygen to the lungs which translate into more oxygen to the brain including those that are in the process of healing. Yogic relaxation increases blood flow to the peripheral organs of the body. Yogic practices also increases haemoglobin therefore oxygen carrying capacity of blood is enhanced.
7. **Improves joint health:** The regular practicing yogic regimen increases joint health and prevent rheumatoid and osteoarthritis. Yoga maintains the flexibility and strength of joints.

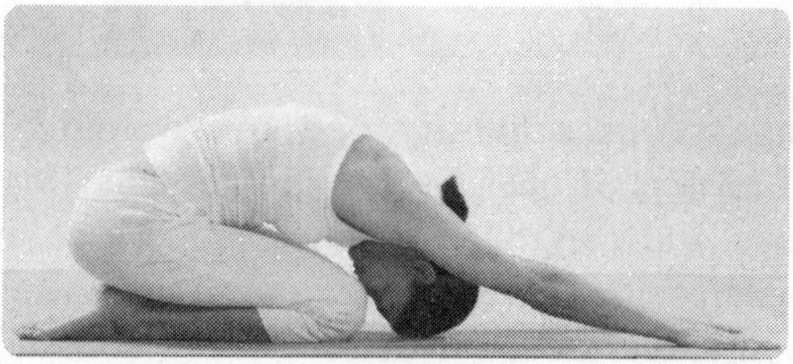

8. **Strengthen bones:** Osteoporosis is a disease of bones that occurs when the body loses too much bone and makes too little bone, or both. As a result, bones become weak and may break from a fall or, in serious cases, from sneezing or minor bumps. Regular practicing of yoga strengthens spine and hip bone density which is usually a problem of geriatric patients or old age persons. There are many scientific evidences which supports that practicing yoga increases the bone density and prevent osteoporosis.
9. **Lowering the risk of CAD:** Coronary artery disease (CAD) occurs by the building of plaque in the arteries of the heart. This condition is called as Atherosclerosis. The arteries become narrow and do not allow oxygen-rich blood flow to the heart. We called it as heart blockage. Pranayam and asana can prevent atherosclerosis. Pranayama shows excellent improvement in the function of heart. Pranayama will remove your heart blockages without spending money. Thirty minutes pranayama daily keeps your heart healthy. People, who

want to prevent heart problems without spending on costly medicines should practice pranayama and yogasana such as Uttanapadasana; Pavanamuktasan and Shavasana.

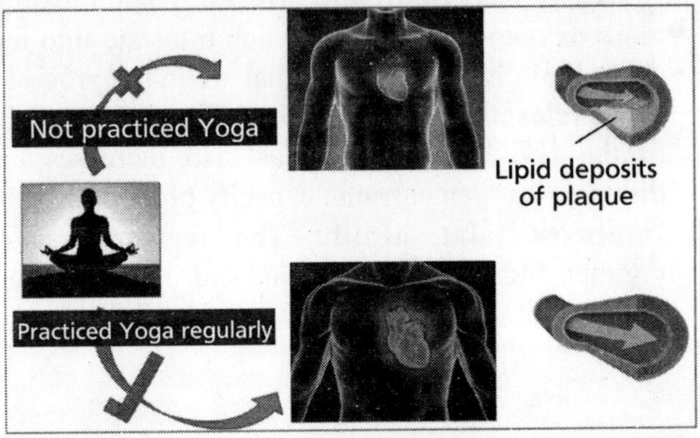

10. **Yoga reduces obesity and overweight:** Yoga works on all aspects of obesity or excess weight. Regular practice of Yoga and controlled lifestyle reduces obesity. It makes a human being agile, efficient and slim. It is suitable for people in any age group. It helps achieve control over mind and behaviour. One can easily control food habits and change lifestyle to reduce the obesity. Yoga has different effect on obesity, which is permanent in nature than other techniques for obesity reduction. There are many scientific reports which demonstrate that yoga fights obesity and overweight.

Health consequences of overweight and obesity

- Obstructive sleep apnea
- Snoring
- Coronary artery disease
- High blood cholesterol
- Type 2 diabetes
- Cancer
- Arthritis
- Stroke
- High blood pressure
- Hypertension
- Excessive sweating

- Liver cirrhosis
- Low back pain
- Gout
- Varicose veins

11. **Improves function of nervous system:** Regular practicing of yoga may help improve your physical and mental well-being. One of the key benefits of yoga lies in its ability to positively impact your nervous system, which may help you develop a healthier stress response. Restorative yoga poses and breathing practices activate parasympathetic nervous system, which can help you handle stress better and invoke feelings of deep relaxation. Neurological disorders like multiple sclerosis, epilepsy. Parkinson's disease and Alzheimer's impact millions world-wide. Yoga practices may impact brain structures and neural networks, as well as the autonomic nervous system, which projects throughout the body. This integration of brain and body systems may be particularly beneficial for those coping with neurological disorders.

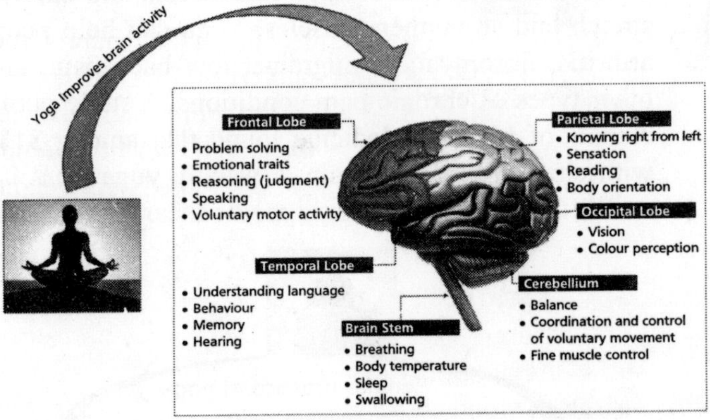

12. **Lowers BP/Hypertension:** Yoga lowers blood pressure naturally by inducing deep relaxation in the body, which is associated with a reduced nervous system activity and a feeling of well-being, probably due to an increase in antioxidants and lower levels of the stress hormone cortisol. High blood pressure is a major risk factor for heart attacks and stroke because blood vessels in the heart or brain are more likely to

rupture under increased pressure. Hypertension is often called the "silent killer" because it is a disease without symptoms until something serious occurs. Yogic Pranayam or breathing is the most efficient way to lower blood pressure.

13. **Improves psychological health:** Practicing yoga regularly improves one's mental health. If you continuously feel that the entire weight of the world's problems is on your shoulders, you might just be following a highly strenuous lifestyle. Yoga helps one soothe their mind as well as their body. Breathing regimes and yoga exercises have been proven to be exceedingly effective in revamping your psychological health by keeping negative elements on the wayside of your life. Five psychological benefits of yoga includes: i) Yoga improves your memory ii) Controls the ravages of traumatic experiences iii) Combating anxiety and depression iv) Keep psychological issues at bay during adolescence v) Improve your overall psychological well-being.
14. **Relieves pain:** Yoga is a mind-body and exercise practice that combines breath control, meditation, and movements to stretch and strengthen muscles. Yoga can help people with arthritis, fibromyalgia, migraine, low back pain, and many other types of chronic pain conditions. A study published in Annals of Internal Medicine found that among 313 people with chronic low back pain, a weekly yoga class increased mobility more than standard medical care for the condition.

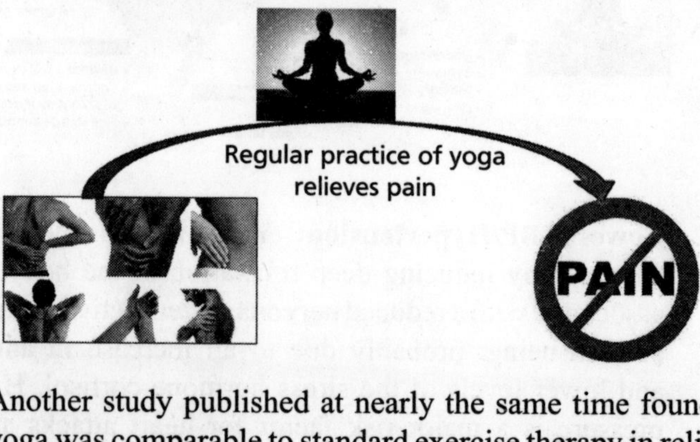

Another study published at nearly the same time found that yoga was comparable to standard exercise therapy in relieving chronic low back pain. A meta-analysis of 17 studies that included more than 1,600 participants concluded that yoga can improve daily function among people with fibromyalgia osteoporosis-related curvature of the spine.

References

1. Mooventhan A & Niventhitha L (2017). Evidence-based effects of yoga in neurological disorders. *Journal of Clinical Neuroscience.*
2. McCall, Timothy. *Yoga as Medicine: The Yogic Prescription for Health and Healing*. NewYork: Bantam, 2007.
3. Khalsa, Sat Bir, Cohen, Lorenzo, McCall, Timothy, Telles, Shirley. *The Principles and Practice of Yoga in Health Care.* Edinburgh: Handspring Publishing, 2016.
4. Payne, Larry, et al. *Yoga Therapy and Integrative Medicine: Where Ancient Science Meets Modern Medicine*. Nashville, TN: Basic Health Publications, Inc., 2015.
5. Edlin, Gordon, and Eric Golanty. *Health and wellness*. Jones & Bartlett Publishers, 2012.
6. Website of American heart association.

❐

Section II

Yoga for Extreme Environment

6
Yoga for Combating the Extreme Cold Environment of Antarctica

Introduction

In the cold environment, ambient temperature of the atmosphere is close to or below 0°C. Antarctica is one of the seven continents with extremely cold climate.

Antarctica contains all areas of land, ice, and sea around the South Pole, extends to the southern polar circle (66° 33' S). Antarctica's ice shield holds approximately 30 million km^2 ice (= 65% of all freshwater resources), which leads to extensive reflection of sunlight. Antarctica's climate is dominated by seasonal changes. Depending on latitude, months of complete darkness in the Antarctic winter alternate with months of 24 h bright daylight in the Antarctic summer. Stays in the Antarctic can be divided into two categories:

Summer expedition: Scientists and workers reside in Antarctic research stations for a time limited to the Antarctic summer using the favorable temperature and light conditions.

Winter-over expedition: During the month of March to September Antarctica has winter condition and scientists and workers reside in the stations year round.

Depending on the nature of stay in Antarctica, inhabitants may have to face great exhaustion, deep cold and dry air, and a different circadian cycle. It has been shown that the environmental changes can lead to hypothermia, changes circadian rhythm, changes in immune system, and changes in hormonal system in humans. The number of inhabitants in Polar Regions is likely to increase, for example, for the extraction of natural resources; therefore knowledge gained in stays in the Antarctic could be used for practical applications. Fig. 1 shows the Indian Antarctic Research Station "Maitri" along with a view of severe blizzard.

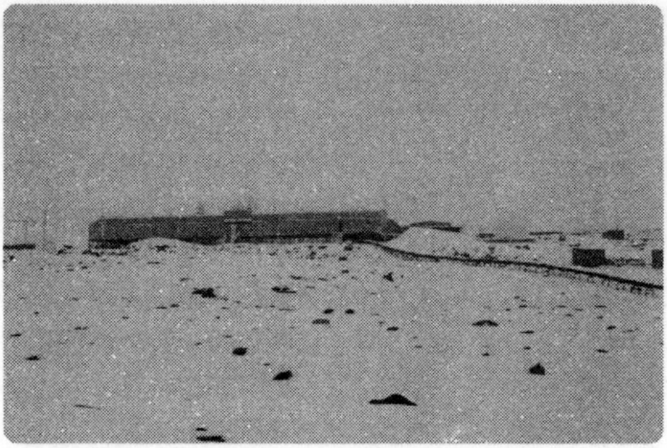

Fig. 1: Indian Antarctic Research Station "Maitri"

Thermoregulation in Cold Environment

Hypothalamus is the thermoregulatory centre which controls the body temperature in human. It receives input from two sets of thermoreceptors:

Receptors in the hypothalamus itself monitors the temperature of the blood as it passes through the brain (the core temperature), and receptors in the skin monitor the external temperature. For appropriate adjustment, both sets of information are needed to the human body. The thermoregulatory centre of hypothalamus sends impulses to several different effectors to adjust body temperature.

The first response to encountering colder condition is voluntary - if too cold, we put extra clothes on - or turn the heating up! It is only when these responses are not enough that the thermoregulatory centre is stimulated. This is part of the autonomic nervous system, so the various responses are all involuntary. When we get too cold, it is the heat conservation centre of the hypothalamus which is stimulated. Note that some of the responses to low temperature actually generate heat (thermogenesis), whilst others just conserve heat.

Thus the human body has a range of responses available, depending on the internal and external temperatures (Brychta and Chen, 2017).

i) Effector response of smooth muscles in arterioles in the skin: Muscles contraction causing vasoconstriction. Less heat is carried from the core to the surface of the body, maintaining core temperature.

ii) Erector response of pili muscles in skin (attached to skin hairs): Muscles contract, raising skin hairs and trapping an insulating layer of still, warm air next to the skin. Not very effective in humans, just causing "goosebumps".

iii) Shivering: Muscles contract and relax repeatedly, generating heat by friction and from metabolic reactions (respiration is only 40% efficient: 60% of increased respiration thus generates heat).

iv) Effector response of adrenal and thyroid glands: Adrenal and thyroid glands secrete adrenaline and thyroxine respectively, which increases the metabolic rate in different tissues, especially the liver, so they work to generate heat.

Antarctic Environment as Space Analogues

Life and work of humans in extreme environments such as the Antarctic can be characterized by the following parameters: They are of high technical dependency (life support, water, climate); there exists great physical and psychological isolation from the usual environment; inhabitants are living and working in a confined space with a small number of unknown individuals and they have to face challenging tasks on site viz. psycho physiological, and cognitive challenges. Risk of failure also exists with high economic and individual loss. There is virtually no possibility for rescue and there is a high necessity to communicate and cooperate within the crew and to the outside individuals. Long-term stay in Antarctica therefore offer an analogy to many conditions encountered in space. The possibility to examine these conditions and their impact on humans as a model for long term space flights, space agencies have incorporated these models into their study program. In general, the study of human physiology in space can be divided into: 1) laboratory and simulation; 2) natural, physical environment; and 3) constructed environment. Although simulation in laboratory are important to prepare space crews for their missions, it is recognized that natural laboratory or space analogue on earth, such as those in polar regions, submarines, and underwater habitats are critical for real-life and real-time observation of human behaviors and experience similar to those in space (Clancey, 2002; Manzey, 2004). As an example, the cold, dry, and radiation condition, as well as difficulty in getting support in remote areas in Antarctica, is suggested to be similar to that in Mars and therefore an ideal testing ground for space crew simulation (Harrison, 1995). Each analogue environment, including Antarctica, offers advantages to study human physiological, psychological and behavioral health in natural setting.

Defence Institute of Physiology and Allied Sciences (DIPAS), Delhi involved in human physiological research in Antarctica, right from the beginning of Antarctic Research of India i.e. way back since 1985. A summary of human physiological research results from the DIPAS Antarctic programmes has been given in Table-1.

Studies of Cold Acclimatization at Antarctica

Understanding the human physiological response in cold is an important military concern. There are several reports of the terrible effects experienced by soldiers during military operations conducted during cold weather. Since, DIPAS is working for military, therefore, understanding the human physiological response in cold is pertinent to develop countermeasures against cold related problems.

A major study into cold adaptation is conducted by DIPAS in Antarctica at the Indian bases (Purkayastha et al. 1997), has conducted this study to assess the status of cold acclimatization (CA) resulting from short and long-term exposure of tropical men to severely cold environment of the Arctic and the Antarctic regions. Five Groups (seven each) of male subjects participated in this study. Cold-induced vasodilatation (CIVD) response was elicited during immersion of the right hand in cold water at 4°C for 30 min at both the Polar Regions to evaluate peripheral CA. The 'standard cold test' at 10 °C for 2 h was administered at the Arctic region on tropical and arctic residents and the data were compared with those for tropical men monitoted at Delhi to ascertain the level of general CA. Group A (control) was studied at Delhi (29°N, 77°E), while Groups B and C were sailed to Antarctica (70°S, 11.5°E). Their CIVD responses were monitored during thirteenth month and seventh to eighth week of stay respectively. There was no deliberate cold exposure, except during their 'occupation demand' outdoor duties. However, outdoor exposure for Group C was more. Group D was airlifted to the Arctic (70°N,

38 °E) and studied during the seventh week of acclimatization. The subjects had regular deliberate cold exposure. For comparison, Group E of arctic residents was studied at the Arctic. Group B did not show any adaptive modification to cold even after a year of sojourn in the Antarctic environment compared to Group A; while Group C subjects, despite their short stay, showed better CIVD response. Group D subjects recorded significant improvement in the response of general cold exposure as well as peripheral vascular response to local cold stress; their responses were comparable to those of the arctic residents (Group E). It is evident that human CA is impossible just by living in the coldest region of the globe even for prolonged periods. Deliberate regular exposure to atmospheric cold is the mandatory factor in developing human CA, the degree of which is related to the intensity of cold exposure.

Effect of Antarctic Environment on Endocrine System

Antarctic harsh environmental condition affects endocrine system. During the Antarctic winter subtle changes in thyroid hormone levels during a winter over stay are related not only to the extreme cold but also to other factors such as physical activity, polar days and polar nights. (Sawhney et al.1995) studied the adaptation of the thyroid gland to the Antarctic environment in nine healthy Indian expedition members of the Sixth Indian Antarctic Expedition during winter over stay at polar latitudes. The circulatory concentrations of thyroid hormones were estimated in New Delhi and during the first week of each month of the stay in Antarctica. At the end of the Austral summer in March, the Total T3 concentrations were found to be significantly lower compared to values recorded in New Delhi and showed a significant increase during the Austral winter in August. The mean TT3 concentrations from May to December were found to be significantly higher than the March or April values. Plasma Total T4 and reverse T3 levels tended to decline in March but remained unaltered during the entire period in Antarctica. The FT4, FT3, TBG and T3 uptake did not show any appreciable change. Though, the TT3:TT4 ratio tended to decline in March and April suggesting decreased peripheral conversion of T4 to T3 as the possible mechanism for a decline in TT3 in March. Physical exertion, harsh weather conditions and prolong exposure to cold appeared to be the major contributory factors. The TSH level in winter months was found to be significantly higher than the base line values. The morning as well as evening cortisol concentrations during the Austral winter were higher than the March values suggesting that cortisol rhythmicity was well maintained in Antarctica, albeit at a higher level. These observations indicated that the subtle changes in thyroid hormones during a prolonged stay at polar latitudes are related not only to the extreme cold but also to other factors such as physical activity, polar days and polar nights. In another study, Malhotra et al. (1998) reported the level of plasma insulin during Antarctic residence. Circulatory levels of insulin were estimated in nine tropical euglycemic men in New Delhi and during the first week of every month of stay in Dakshin Gangotri, Antarctica. The insulin levels during winter months were found to be significantly lower than the base line values. This decline in insulin in Antarctica might be important in increasing substrate availability for heat production by facilitating lipolysis and hepatic glucose output. The study by Sawhney et al. (1998) also reported the Pituitary-gonadal hormones during prolonged residency in Antarctica. In this study, Plasma luteinizing hormone (LH), follicle stimulating hormone (FSH), prolactin (PRL) and testosterone levels were measured in nine eugonadal men in New Delhi and during the 1st week of different months of their stay at Dakshin Gangotri in Antarctica. Plasma testosterone tended to increase in March, but a significant increase ($P < 0.05$) was not seen until April. The mean testosterone levels in May, June, September and November were also significantly higher than the March or base line values. The absolute values of LH, FSH and PRL did not show any month-to-month changes in Antarctica. However, when the hormone levels were expressed as a percentage of the individual annual Antarctic mean, significant differences as a percentage of the individual annual Antarctic mean, significant differences were observed. The testosterone peak in April, May and June was associated with an increase in LH. The nadirs of testosterone, LH, FSH and PRL were seen in either July or August. FSH showed the highest values in March, whereas the highest PRL values were seen in November. These observations suggest the presence of circannual variations in gonadotropin, PRL and LH in Antarctica which are independent of polar days and polar nights. It appears that factors other than the duration of daylight might be involved in regulating these changes. The significance of maintenance of testosterone levels in the supra-physiological range in Antarctica remains unknown but may be important in acclimatization/habituation to the extreme polar cold by increasing basal metabolic rate, protein synthesis and erythropoisis. The study conducted by Harinath et al. (2005) reported about the autonomic nervous system and adrenal response to cold in man at Antarctica. Here the objective was to evaluate the role of the autonomic nervous system and adrenal system in acclimatization to cold in tropical men during short or prolonged sojourns at Antarctica. To fulfill the objective, a study was carried out on volunteers of the 18th winter over team and 19th summer team of an Indian Antarctic Expedition. The summer team members were evaluated at Delhi; during voyage; and on days 7, 30, and 60 of their stay at Antarctica. Identical studies were performed in winter over team members who had stayed at Antarctica for 14 months. The parameters examined included heart rate, blood pressure, oral temperature, index finger skin temperature, heart rate variability, urinary epinephrine and norepinephrine, and salivary cortisol. The results suggested that the resting heart rate and blood pressure in summer team members significantly increased ($P < .05$) on days 7 and 30 of their stay at Antarctica and returned to baseline Delhi values by day 60. The index finger temperature declined ($P < .05$) on day 7 at Antarctica and remained at lower levels during the entire period of observations. Heart rate variability showed an imbalance of autonomic nervous system effects with predominance of low-frequency band on day 7 of stay and returned to Delhi values by day 60. The urinary excretion of epinephrine and nor-epinephrine and salivary Cortisol were also increased on day 7 and declined to baseline Delhi values after 2 months of stay. Compared with the ST group, the winter over team group showed a significantly higher ($P < .05$) resting heart rate, blood pressure, and low-frequency power and urinary excretion of nor-epinephrine. The study concluded that Antarctic residency during austral summer results in gradual attenuation of sympathetic tone and a shift of autonomic balance toward the parasympathetic side. However, winter over team members showed a predominance of sympathetic and adrenal activity compared with initial responses of summer team members, suggesting deconditioning or possible resetting of the autonomic nervous system.

Appetite and Neuronal Peptides

Early expeditions led by Scott, Shackleton and Mawson drew attention to the harsh realities of living in Antarctica and many of these men suffered from diet-related problems, compounded by stresses already being experienced in conditions of extreme cold and physical exhaustion (Taylor 1992).

Although most bases are now equipped with more than adequate food supplies even as far inland as the South Pole, there are still issues associated with maintaining the food provided to isolated field groups. The main concern for these field events is that they may have to cope for long periods without re-supply so the food they take must be preserved, and remain useable after several months. Field rations also need to be durable in order to handle exposure to a broad potential temperature range over the summer field season, which could subject the food to many freeze-thaw cycles. As the availability of fresh food is very limited for winter-over personnel, vitamin and mineral deficiencies can begin to develop in personnel. Though, the food eaten on bases in Antarctica is very similar to the food that we eat at home, of course. The biggest deficiency is in the supply of fresh fruit and vegetables - i.e. there aren't any for most of the time, only when a ship comes in or an aircraft lands. This means that for much of the year the food is frozen, dried or tinned. Modern techniques in food preservation and fortification mean that there is no danger of suffering from a deficiency disease, Therefore, due to the non-availability of fresh food the dietary stress is also experienced by the expeditioners. Vats et al. (2005) performed a study on Appetite regulatory peptides in Indian Antarctic summer expedition members. The study reported the changes in appetite regulatory peptides i.e. leptin and neuropeptide Y in relation to energy intake and expenditure of the Antarctic expeditioners. (Vats et al. 2007) further reported the Changes in vitamin status of Indian Antarctic expeditioners during a one-month stay in Austral Summer. Vitamin C levels decreased significantly (P< .001) after one month stay in Antarctica compared with basal values (1.31 +/-0.076 mg/dL during phase I to 0.81+/-0.063 mg/dL during phase III). However, these levels were still within the normal reference range. Therefore, this study found no water-soluble vitamin deficiencies in participants consuming processed and canned food after 1 month in Antarctica. The summer expedition members do not face the absence of sunlight of Antarctic continent while winter members spent few months without exposing to sunlight therefore vitamin status in winter team member may also be decreased as compared to summer members though the data was not observed.

Antarctica Environment and Sleep

The circadian rhythm — the variation of various body functions over the time course of a day — is a ubiquitous phenomenon (Reid and Zee, 2009). Hypothalamus and in particular the area of the suprachiasmatic nucleus (SCN) are key locations in regulation of circadian rhythm. The role of sleep and circadian phase on safety, performance and psychological health during expeditions is very important aspect of biomedical research. Bhattacharyya et al. (2008) have studied the changes in sleep patterns during prolonged stays in Antarctica. In this study, the changes in sleep patterns of six members of the Indian expedition team during their winter stay at Indian research base Maitri, Antarctica were studied. Total sleep time was decreased in the expedition members during Antarctic stay as compared to Delhi baseline values in all months, sleep efficiency decreased significantly during winter months, duration of waking period after sleep onset increased significantly in winter, sleep latency increased immediately after exposure in January, slow wave sleep reduced during dark winter months, whereas rapid eye movement sleep increased during dark winter months. This study observed a prevailing general trend of sleep disturbances among winter over expedition members during their stay at Maitri station in Antarctica.

Human Immune System

The immune system is one of the major thrust areas in understanding the effects of adverse climatic conditions on human health. A study was conducted by DIPAS, Delhi for evaluation of effect of harsh environment on immune response of summer and winter team members of the 28th Indian Antarctic expedition.

Summer Expedition: Summer team member reached Antarctic research stations of India (Maitri and Bharti) by ship from Capetown. During the voyage many of the expeditioners were affected by seasickness. Effects of ship borne journey and the impact of Antarctic harsh environment on serum immunoglobulin (IgG,

IgM, IgA) levels and their relationship with seasickness in Indian expeditioners indicated that — one month onboard ship journey induced an increase in serum IgA levels and decrease in IgG levels while after being one month off board at the Indian research station Maitri, the levels remained same. Moreover, serum IgG level showed a positive correlation with seasickness whereas IgA level showed a negative correlation. IgM levels were not altered in comparison to the base line control. Thus, the study concluded that ship borne journey and Antarctic environment lead to increased serum IgA levels (Mishra *et al.,* 2011). Furthermore, the study on mucosal immunity by analysing saliva suggested that ship borne journey and Antarctic environment increased the SIgA (salivary IgA) levels while that of SIgM level was not altered on-board but decreased by staying for one month at Antarctica. No significant alteration was found in the serum TGF-β and cortisol level at any point of time. Thus it can be concluded that ship borne journey and Antarctic environment may induce the SIgA level while SIgM level decreased in environmental extremes of Antarctica (Mishra *et al.,* 2012). It is also suggested that since both serum and saliva IgA levels were enhanced throughout, therefore could be a possible biomarker for environmental stress. The data observed on cytokine profiling confirmed that ship-borne journey induced an increase in TNF-α, IFN-γ, and B cell activating factor (BAFF) levels while moderate decreases in TGF-β and cortisol levels in human serum. However, after being off board for one month at Maitri station, levels of above cytokines, cortisol and BAFF were decreased but MIP-1α was significantly increased. This data for the first time suggests that tremendous stress during ship-borne journey to the Antarctica eventually resulted in increased TH1-biased immunity (Mishra *et al.,* 2010).

Winter Expedition: The study was also performed on winter team members which suggest that TNF-α and MIP-1α levels were significantly increased in March, May and August months, while IFN-γ levels were increased in March and May. TGF-β levels showed a significant decrease in March and May. Serum IgA levels were significantly increased during the entire period of the stressful expedition suggesting again that serum IgA could be a potential biomarker even for extreme environmental conditions (Yadav *et al.,* 2012). We have also reported that one month ship borne journey did not cause any significant change in the sHLA-G level as compared to the baseline level of the summer expeditioners. sHLA-G levels were not changed significantly in the months of March, May, August and November as compared to the baseline level of the winter expeditioners (Mishra *et al.*, 2014). The study of complement system indicated that complement C3 up-regulated during ship journey and during peak winter in August (Yadav *et al.,* 2015). Study has also reported the evidence for altered metabolic pathways during Antarctic stay by (1) H-NMR spectroscopy based metabolomics and clinical studies on subjects of sea-voyage and Antarctic-stay, indicating the significant change in the metabolism of the expeditioners (Yadav *et al.,* 2014). The study conducted on Antarctic sojourners indicated that extreme climatic conditions affect human system.

Yoga for Better Acclimatization to Antarctic Environment

The Antarctica is the coldest place to live, in summer the temperature is around 0°C but as winter approaches the temperature dip down to –20 to –40°C or even more and our bodies begin to feel the winter enduring effects, the importance of maintaining healthy cycles, adjusting to changes in environment becomes more obvious. Yoga could be one of the way, we can choose to build health and vitality through practices.

Cold environment often creates tension and tight muscles often resulting in postural effects. The coldness of Antarctic weather causes muscles to contract. Asana and pranayama practices that heat the body help to maintain elasticity of the muscles and mobility of the joints, relieving cramps and soreness. Fig. 2. Shows yoga being performed at Antarctica by Indian expedition members.

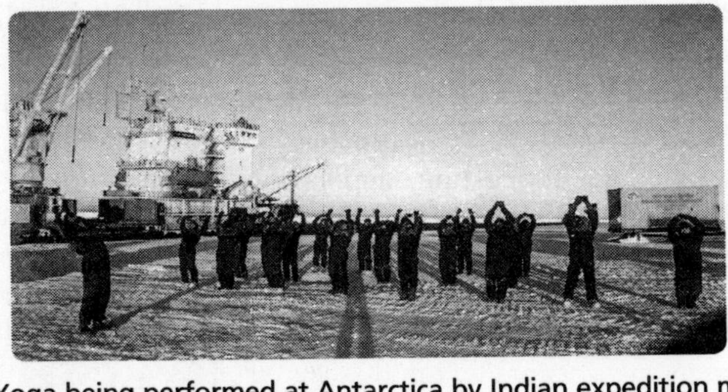

Fig. 2: Yoga being performed at Antarctica by Indian expedition members

Since Antarctic winter-over personnel do not expose to sunlight for several months, it results in low energy levels, feelings of fatigue, sluggishness and the urge to hibernate. Because the heat the body generates from the sun helps to relax muscles, soothe the mind and maintain healthy sleep patterns. Pranayama practices and asana internally heat the body leaving skin and muscular tissues much more elastic. Consistent yoga practice make energized, in general and throughout the winter, can help provide consistent energy levels.

Yoga improves our energy because it improves the functioning of our pancreas, which regulates our insulin levels, therefore regulating the blood-sugar levels and our energy. Yogic practices also make joints flexible during which synovial fluid is released within the joint, which acts as a lubricant. This creates smoother movements, increased & maintained range of motion within the joints.

Ujjayi pranayama which leads to restore internal energy is a very gentle tightening of the back of the throat, breath moves freely in and out through the nostrils. Through slight muscular contraction, Ujjayi breath increases the core temperature of the body aiding the process of detoxification throughout our practice. This practice actively cleanses the lungs of mucus and increases the amount of freshly oxygenated blood flowing throughout the body, improving overall circulation. Ujjayi pranayama not only heats the body but it also helps to soothe and calm the mind. Tension from cold and damp weather does not just take a physical toll but can be mentally taxing as well.

Conclusion

Antarctic environment has the ability to place the human body under increased physical and psychological stress. People have overcome the majority of challenges presented by living conditions in Antarctica either through micro-scale modification of their environment using clothing and shelter or by yoga for physiological adaptation to the environment. Overall, Yoga practice will preventatively support the body, reducing congestion, supporting the respiratory system, invigorating metabolism and strengthening immune system in order to combat Antarctic extreme cold induced illnesses.

Table 1. Summary of studies of Antarctic environment on human physiological responses

S.N.	Physiological observations	References
1.	Thyroid function during a prolonged stay in Antarctica.	Sawhney *et al.*, 1995
2.	Cold acclimatization of tropical men during short & long term sojourn to polar environments.	Purkayastha *et al.*, 1997
3.	Pituitary-gonadal hormones during prolonged residency in Antarctica.	Sawhney *et al.*, 1997
4.	Plasma insulin and growth hormone during Antarctic residence.	Malhotra *et al.*, 1998
5.	Autonomic nervous system and adrenal response to cold in man at Antarctica.	Harinath *et al.*, 2005
6.	Appetite regulatory peptides in Indian Antarctic expeditioners.	Vats *et al.*, 2005
7.	Changes in vitamin status of Indian Antarctic expeditioners during a one-month stay in Austral Summer.	Vats *et al.*, 2007
8.	Changes in sleep patterns during prolonged stays in Antarctica.	Bhattacharya *et al.*, 2008
9.	Ship-borne journey induces Th1 cytokines level in Antarctic summer expeditioners.	Mishra *et al.*, 2010
10.	Serum levels of immunoglobulins (IgG, IgA, IgM) in Antarctic summer expeditioners and their relationship with seasickness.	Mishra *et al.*, 2011
11.	Antarctic harsh environment as natural stress model: Impact on mucosal immunity.	Mishra *et al.*, 2012
12.	Winter-over expedition in Antarctica: Impact on immune system.	Yadav *et al.*, 2012

13.	Effect of extreme conditions of Antarctica on human leukocyte antigen-G in Indian expeditioners.	Mishra *et al.,* 2014
14.	Evidence for altered metabolic pathways during environmental stress: (1) H-NMR spectroscopy based metabolomics and clinical studies on subjects of sea-voyage and Antarctic-stay.	Yadav *et al.,* 2014
15.	Activation of complement system during ship voyage and winter-over expedition in Antarctica.	Yadav *et al.,* 2015

References

1. Akita S, Conn PM, Melmed S. Leukemia inhibitory factor (LIF) induces acute adrenocorticotrophic hormone (ACTH) secretion in fetal rhesus macaque primates: a novel dynamic test of pituitary function. J. Clin. Endocrinol. Metab., 1996, 81, 4170-78.
2. Besedovsky HO, Del Rey A, Sorkin E, Dinarello CA. Immunoregulatory feedback between interleukin-1 and glucocorticoid hormones. Science., 1986, 233, 652-54.
3. Bhattacharyya M, Pal MS, Sharma YK, Majumdar D. Changes in sleep patterns during prolonged stays in Antarctica.Int J Biometeorol. 2008 Nov; 52(8):869-79.
4. Brychta RJ, Chen KY. Cold-induced thermogenesis in humans. Eur J Clin Nutr. 2017; 71(3): 345-352.
5. Chrousos GP. The hypothalamic–pituitary–adrenal axis and immune-mediated inflammation. New Engl. J. Med., 1995, 332, 1351-62.
6. Clancey WJ. A framework for analog studies of Mars surface operation: Using the flash line Mars Arctic Research Station, USA, NASA/AMES Research Center, 2002, 1-18.
7. Harinath K, Malhotra AS, Pal K, Prasad R, Kumar R, Sawhney RC. Autonomic nervous system and adrenal response to cold in man at Antarctica. Wilderness Environ Med. 2005 Summer;16 (2): 81-91.

8. Harrison, A.A. Antarctica: prototype for outer space (NASA-TM-108095). Scott Polar Research Institute, University of Cambridge, 1995, 1-13.
9. Kovacs, K.J. & Elenkov, I.J. Differential dependence of ACTH secretion induced by various cytokines on the integrity of the paraventricular nucleus. J. Neuroendocrinol., 1995, 7, 15-23.
10. Malhotra AS, Pal K, Prasad R, Bajaj AC, Kumar R, Sawhney RC. Plasma insulin and growth hormone during antarctic residence. Jpn J Physiol. 1998 Apr;48(2):167-9.
11. Manzey D. Human missions to Mars: new psychological challenges and research issues. Acta Astronaut, 2004, 33 (3-9), 781-90.
12. Mishra KP,Yadav AP, Lilly Ganju. Antarctic harsh environment as natural stress model: Impact on mucosal immunity. Indian Journal of clinical Biochemistry Ind J Clin Biochem. DOI 10.1007/s12291-012-0213-z
13. Mishra KP, Yadav AP, Shweta, Chanda S, Ganju L, Majumdar D, Ilavazhagan G. Ship-borne journey induces Th1 cytokines level in antarctic summer expeditioners. Immunol Invest. 2010; 39 (7): 770-9.
14. Mishra KP, Yadav AP, Shweta, Chanda S, Majumdar D, Ganju L. Serum levels of immunoglobulins (IgG, IgA, IgM) in Antarctic summer expeditioners and their relationship with seasickness. Cell Immunol. 2011;271(1):29-35.
15. Mishra KP, Yadav AP, Sharma YK, Ganju L, Singh SB. Effect of extreme conditions of Antarctica on human leukocyte antigen-G in Indian expeditioners. Indian J Med Res. 2014 Oct; 140(4):520-3.
16. Purkayastha SS, Majumdar D, Selvamurthy W. Cold Acclimatization of Tropical Men during Short & Long term Sojourn to Polar Environments. Defence Science Journal. 1997; 47: 149-158.
17. Reid KJ, Zee, PC. Circadian rhythm disorder. Semin Neurol 2009; 29: 393-405.
18. Sawhney RC, Malhotra AS, Nair CS, Bajaj AC, Rajan KC, Pal K, Prasad R, Basu M.Thyroid function during a prolonged stay in Antarctica. Eur J Appl Physiol Occup Physiol. 1995; 72 (1-2): 127-33.

19. Sawhney RC, Malhotra AS, Prasad R, Pal K, Kumar R, Bajaj AC. Pituitary-gonadal hormones during prolonged residency in Antarctica.Int J Biometeorol. 1998; 42 (1): 51-4.
20. Taylor, D. M. 1992 Modification of the type of dietary fat at an Antarctic station: impact on cardiovascular risk factors, Kingston Tasmania: Antarctic Division, Dept. of the Arts, Sport, The Environment and Territories.
21. Vats P, Singh SN, Singh VK, Shyam R, Upadhyay TN, Singh SB, Banerjee PK. Appetite regulatory peptides in Indian Antarctic expeditioners. Nutr Neurosci. 2005; 8(4): 233-8.
22. Vats P, Singh SN, Singh VK, Shyam R, Upadhyay TN, Singh SB, Banerjee PK. Changes in vitamin status of Indian Antarctic expeditioners during a one-month stay in Austral Summer. Wilderness Environ Med. 2007 Winter;18 (4):258-63.
23. Yadav AP, Mishra KP, Ganju Lilly, Singh SB. Winter-over expedition in Antarctica: Impact on immune system. Neuroimmunomodulation. 2012;19(6):327-33.
24. Yadav AP, Chaturvedi S, Mishra KP, Pal S, Ganju L, Singh SB. Evidence for altered metabolic pathways during environmental stress: (1)H-NMR spectroscopy based metabolomics and clinical studies on subjects of sea-voyage and Antarctic-stay. Physiol Behav. 2014 Aug;135:81-90.
25. Yadav AP, Mishra KP, Tanwar H, Sharma NK, Singh SB and Ganju L. Activation of complement system during ship voyage and winter-over expedition in Antarctica. J Marine Sc Res & Development, 2015, 5:3, 1-8.

❐

7

High Altitude Environment and Yoga for Better Acclimatization

Yoga is for the spiritual development of everyone, irrespective of age, caste, creed or sex. It is universal. Defence Institute of Physiology and Allied Sciences (DIPAS) has given a scientific outlook on yoga, with particular reference to the armed forces. Armed forces have accepted the introduction of yoga, and the National Defence directed training is already underway. A customized yoga package for high altitude has already been given to the armed forces for training programs, which is complementing the present physical training program. It is a huge program, with a large number of people to be trained throughout the country. DIPAS conduct training programs of a high level to train our armed forces instructors, and these trained inspectors implement the yogic exercises for armed force personnel at their unit.

A lot of research has been conducted at DIPAS in the last three decades where different forms of the yoga were evaluated scientifically. DIPAS has extensively worked on stressful environmental conditions and made soldiers life easier by yogic practices. Stress can be physical, environmental, psychological or emotional, and how yoga can be used as an important method of coping with the mechanism of stress is important to understand. Stress can originate in the physical environment such as soldiers sitting on the snow-clad mountains of the Siachen glacier where they are exposed to the physical extremes of high altitude and hypoxia. They are also exposed to the psychological stresses of isolation, monotony, separation from family, with shelling, at times, coming from across the border. In this way they are exposed to both physical and environmental extremes.

High Altitude: High altitude has no exact definition but the height above sea level, where alterations in human physiology begin, affect the physical performance and produce pathological changes related to lack of oxygen is defined as high altitude. High altitude is divided into three categories:

1. High altitude (2500-3500 metres): Altitude illness common with rapid ascent
2. Very high altitude (3500-5800 metres): Altitude illness common. Arterial oxygen saturation < 90%. Marked hypoxemia during exercise.
3. Extreme altitude (>5800 metres): Marked hypoxemia at rest. Progressive deterioration, despite maximal acclimatization. Permanent survival cannot be maintained.

Human Physiology at High Altitude

When a person is acutely exposed to high altitude (above 5000 m), shortly, in minutes after such an acute exposure, a significant drop in oxygen saturation (SaO_2), the concentration of oxygen in the blood occurs, which is approximately 95% and 100% at sea level which decreased to ~75%. If the person is continuously staying in the following days the SaO_2 will increase back to ~85% as a result of successful acclimatization. Usually blood oxygen levels should remain >80%, otherwise organ function of the brain and heart might be altered. Concomitantly with the drop in SaO_2, as one of the acclimatization processes, ventilation will be nearly doubled at altitude as compared to sea level, known as hyperventilation. This will lead to lower alveolar CO_2 concentration, thereby increasing the level of oxygen in lungs. The reduced CO_2 concentration in the lungs will attenuate the acid base balance, leading to alkalosis. This alkalosis triggers an increased bicarbonate excretion via kidney in following days to normalize the pH of blood. Besides hyperventilation, the autonomic nervous system will stimulate cardiovascular response, which includes an increase in heart rate and blood pressure as well as erythropoiesis, triggered by increased erythropoietin (EPO) production and release. The enhanced EPO level causes increased red blood cells and hemoglobin (Hb) concentration, leading to higher oxygen transport capacity of blood.

It has been found that an increase of Hb by 3g/l leads to an increase of about 1% in VO2 max. The carotid body plays an important role in sensing the change in the arterial oxygen partial pressure. The changes are mediated to the brainstem via signal processing in which the hypoxia inducible factor (HIF) is involved. It increases (i) a hypoxic ventilator response (HVR) of the lungs and (ii) cardiac output by increasing heart rate. Above 5500 m, regardless of how long and smooth the acclimatization process might be, no acclimatization will be possible. Table 1 summarizes the risk factors, clinical features, and preventive strategies for high altitude illnesses.

Table 1: High altitude illnesses

Condition	Excerbating factors	Clinical features	Prevention
Acute mountain sickness (AMS)	Previous altitude sickness, Rapid ascent, Excessive training early in acclimatization period	Presence of headache and one or more of the following: Gastrointestinal e.g. anorexia, nausea, vomiting - Fatigue or weakness - Dizziness or lightheadedness- - Difficulty in sleeping	Ascent rate (<300 m per day with rest day every 1000 m), Avoid ascent with symptoms, Yoga practice for high altitude hypoxia.
High altitude cerebral edema (HACE)	Previous altitude sickness; Rapid ascent; Excessive training early in acclimatization period	Change in mental status or ataxia in person with AMS or Change in mental status and ataxia in person without AMS Other features: Irrationality, diplopia, hallucinations, papilloedema, tachycardia, tachypnoea, cyanosis.	Early recognition and management of symptoms of AMS
High altitude pulmonary edema (HAPE)	Rapid ascent; Pulmonary hypertension; Congestive heart failure; Chronic obstructive pulmonary disease; Absence of single pulmonary artery; Brisk hypoxic pulmonary vasoconstrictor response; Excessive physical exertion and cold; Respiratory tract infection	Presence of two of the following signs: Crackles/wheeze in at least 1 lung field; Central cyanosis; Tachypnoea; Tachycardia and Presence of Dyspnoea at rest and Cough (dry/productive); Reduced exercise tolerance or fatigue; Chest tightness. Other features: - ECG: right ventricular strain; CXR: prominent pulmonary vessels and patchy infiltrate	Ascent rate (<300 m per day with rest day every 1000 m); Avoid overexertion;

Yoga as a Stress Buster

The internal origins of stress are psychological and emotional in nature. Whatever the source of stress may be it still has two components: stress which has a positive value and distress which has a negative value. The positive element should lead to creativity. So how can stress be kept within optimum limits in an organization such as the armed forces? This is where the DIPAS's primary objective of stress management is focused, and doing research in the area of yoga and stress management.

If stress management with an overall social dimension will not be taken care, it will merely lead to an exaggerated arousal of the body and mind which will ultimately lead to a deterioration of performance in life, as in the case of stress-induced disorders such as hypertension, coronary artery diseases and diabetes. There is a whole spectrum of diseases related to stress-induced problems. So how can yoga help us to maintain the positive dimension of stress, to endure a level of stress without allowing it to manifest within negative dimensions?

There are many studies which reported focused perception. Even though in yoga we have three levels of perception it is our attitude towards the perception of stress on those levels that is of primary importance. If a person does not perceive a factor within a situation as stressful then it is not stressful. How can a person moderate his attitudes, values, personality traits to react to stress constructively, to recognize the stress for what it is?

The first step towards stress management is to moderate the perception of the level of stress by the entire level of the brain, the cerebrum, the cortex, the association memory (which keeps all the learning experiences from childhood). Even though there is a genetic component which cannot be altered very much, a major component of the learning experience can be regulated to a large extent. So the first step towards the management of stress is to moderate the quality of perception.

Once a person has rated a stress at a particular level, his reaction is then dependent on the quality of his perception. As these behavioural reactions are both physical and psychological they are amenable to moderation by yogic practices. Yoga does not mean just practising a few asanas and pranayamas, rather it has to become a discipline and a way of life.

On these two levels how do the yoga practices help to moderate our reactions to stress? By harmonizing the sympathetic and parasympathetic activity, regulation of heart rate, blood pressure, sugar levels etc. is enhanced, and the whole physical infrastructure becomes a more efficient and stronger medium for performance at level one and two. The third level of stress management in yoga is stress release. Yoga helps with the management of experiential stress on all the three levels of perception. Yoga helps to relax and decreases anxiety and stress. When you relax and slow the pace of your breath, the pace of mind is calmed and quieted.

Effects of Yoga Training at High Altitude

A study reported by Himashree et al. (2016) suggested that practice of yoga facilitates improvements in health and performance at high altitude and is superior to routine training with physical exercises. Comprehensive yogic practices are an effective modality for improving health and performance at high altitude. High altitude is a psychophysiological stress for natives of lower altitudes. In this study, 200 soldiers took part in the study. The yoga group showed a significant improvement in health indices and performance as compared with the control group. They had lower weights, Body Fat Percentage (BFP), Respiratory Rate (RR), Diastolic Blood Pressure (DBP), and anxiety scores. They also had a significantly higher EtCO2, forced vital capacity, forced expiratory volume in the first second (FEV1), and VO2 Max. Also, the yoga group showed a significant reduction in serum cholesterol, low-density lipoprotein, triglycerides, and blood urea as compared with their pre-yoga levels and with the exercise group reported with varied results (Himashree *et al.,* 2016).

Defence Institute of Physiology and Allied Sciences (DIPAS) has conducted a series of research projects to explore the prophylactic, promotive and curative potentials of yoga with particular reference to its application for the armed forces since last 30 years. These studies were conducted on the soldiers who practiced a battery of yogic practices including Asanas, Pranayamaand Meditation and on people who have been practicing it for years. The research studies showed that yogic practices helps to achieve a better autonomic balance, orthostatic tolerance, relative hypo-metabolic state and thermoregulatory efficiency to cold stress. Yoga has been shown to improve almost all aspects of physiological performance and efficiency across different ages. These scientific studies have helped to a great extent to formulate yoga packages for the armed forces (Saha *et al.,* 2015).

It has been reported (Ray *et al.,* 1983; 1986; 2001a; 2001b; 2011) that physical and cognitive performance improved in terms of oxygen consumption, flexibility, anaerobic threshold, strength through yogic practice. Physiological responses were recorded at 10°C on the yoga participants (Selvamurthy *et al.,* 1988).

In addition to that DIPAS has made yogic modules for optimization of performance at high altitude through yogic practice. Contributions are also made at a molecular level of physical and cognitive performance improvement through yogic practice. Yogic practice has the beneficial role to prevent age related degenerative changes in the oxygen metabolism, antioxidants redox status (Pal *et al.,* 2013). Ray et.al have shown that at high altitude, after 4 days of continuous strenuous military operation subjects who were practicing yoga for 6 months had better recovery heart rate after exercise, improved VO2max as compared to those who followed usual physical training programme. A number of experiments on yoga were conducted by DIPAS. In a study, DIPAS conducted experiment on two groups [i. physical training group (control) and ii. yoga training group (experimental)], for over a period of six months. In the experimental group (i.e. yoga training) it was found that the autonomic equilibrium between the sympathetic and parasympathetic nervous systems was altered. The parasympathetic tone had a gradual build-up (after comparing the cardiovascular response, heart rate, the pressure at systolic and diastolic level between both groups) which is very vital. During stress, one needs the activation of the excitatory system (the sympathetic system) and when stress is removed there is a need to restore equilibrium (the inhibitory or parasympathetic system). Over the six month period, the soldiers practising *yoga sadhana* had a very low pulse rate of about 50, 55 or 60.

The physical conditioning of *yoga sadhana* has two main advantages. One is to create very high inhibitory tone and the other is to optimize temporary reaction to stress (i.e. sympathetic reaction or arousal to stress whether it be emotional, physical or environmental). So the research indicates that *yoga sadhana* modulates and optimizes sympathetic activity in the stress situation and immediately restores equilibrium, so that the situation no longer demands or requires stress control by the intervention of the inhibitory parasympathetic system. So study indicated that with *yoga sadhana* there is a gradual build-up of inhibitory tone or parasympathetic tone, and heart rate, systolic and diastolic blood pressure tend to show a fall.

Yoga builds up the vehicle tone of the sympathetic and parasympathetic responses. It also cultivates energy conservation so the body functions from a more equilibrated state. Energy is not wasted and performance is enhanced. During times of rest, energy conservation is optimized so that reserves are built up which can otherwise become over depleted during times of stress.

Prana is of vital importance here. The starting point of regulation of *prana* is respiration, i.e. breathing. If we can synchronize, modulate, regulate our breathing then we can attain this equilibrated state. That is why yogis have a very low breathing rate of four to six breaths per minute, whereas ours may be about eighteen, twenty or twenty-two breaths per minute. So even if ordinary people like us can do yoga sadhana for just six months there is a tendency for the breath rate to decrease. The rate decreases but ventilation remains optimized, so this lower rate of breathing is more economical but not at the expense of ventilation (Joshi *et al.,* 1992).

When we are in states of anxiety, under tension and pressure, we will have a very high frequency wave which has a low amplitude. However, once we start to relax this will shift towards a lower frequency and higher amplitude. In the experimental group (yoga), over the six month period, there was a gradual build-up, and even a resting level of alpha activity indicating a state of mental tranquility and brain synchronization.

At the Siachen base camp a study was conducted by DIPAS, with the control group and the experimental group (yoga). The tendency was to lose body heat due to the environment. After six months of asana and pranayama practice the yogic group was able to sustain a higher core temperature. This can be achieved either by heat conservation or by generating more heat to compensate for the loss. The blood flow to the skin was examined. In both groups this difference was insignificant, which suggested that the inner core temperature maintenance is sustained by heat production rather than by heat conservation.

Study also looked into the electro-myographic factor and reported that shivering started much later in the yogic group and was also of a lower magnitude, suggesting that heat production was achieved by non-shivering thermogenesis, i.e. the metabolic means of heat production which does not use energy but only substrate and hormones that are available in the body. Yoga practices help to tone up non-shivering thermogenesis as is evident from the fact that the shivering response manifested much later and was much milder in the yoga group than the physical training group. Even six months of *yogasana* practice showed a definite improvement in tolerance to cold.

Body flexibility forms an integral part of physical fitness. After six months with both groups study reported equal achievement with some components and found total flexion in all joints. However, with the experimental group, it was reported that regular yoga practice can improve the flexibility of various musculature systems even if begun after middle age, 40–45 years.

Psychological functions of study participants were also examined. Yoga is not just the practice of asanas, if the mind is not involved an aspect of the asana has been lost and it is no longer yoga. The spin off from doing each asana with mental concentration is improved learning efficiency, memory, determination and better psychomotor performance. Parameters were measured by using psychological instruments which distinguished between simple reaction, super reaction and changed reaction. Improvement was found in yoga practitioner particularly in the area of learning efficiency.

Yoga also serves as a prophylactic against certain diseases. If we take any one disease, we can attribute it to any one of five factors: lack of exercise; disharmony between body and mind; stress due to occupational and social demands; pollution; and infection. Yoga can protect against these five hazards by forming a pattern of complete exercise. It tones up the muscular and skeletal system and massages the internal organs to activate both the neural and endocrine systems. It brings harmony between mind and body, modulates the stress response and one's attitude to the stress, tones up the nervous system, strengthens the detoxifying systems to handle pollutants and toxic substances effectively, and fortifies the immune system. It also has a curative effect on some of the psychosomatic disorders such as hypertension and diabetes. It is a complete physiological and psychological exercise.

One may wonder how yoga can affect all these responses. The practice of asanas may send a volley of nerve impulses from muscles and joints, spine and other receptors located on the surface as well as inside the viscera. It can influence the haemo-dynamic mechanisms, improving blood circulation to vital organs. It may also act through the neuro-endocrine axis. Yoga is an effective system of preventive health, and scientific evidence in support of this concept is fast emerging. In conclusion, we can say, the practice of yoga facilitates improvements in health and performance at high altitude and is superior to routine training with physical exercises.

Special Yoga Package for High Altitude

(A) Universal Prayer

(B) Loosening Exercise (while seated in)

Sukhasana (Easy Pose)

Procedure

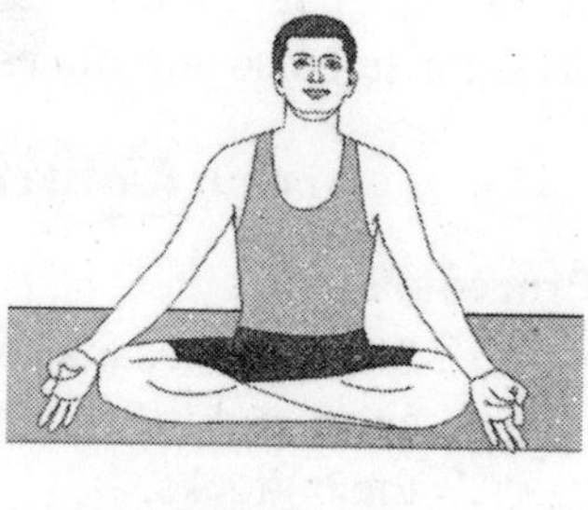

1. Sit with the legs straight in front of the body.
2. Bend one leg and place the foot under the opposite thigh.
3. Bend the other leg and place the foot under the opposite thigh.
4. Place the hands on the knees in *gyana mudra.*
5. Without straining keep the head, neck and back upright and straight. Relax the whole body.

Benefits: Helps mental and physical balance without causing any strain in the body.

- Hand Stretch Parallel to the Ground:
- Hand Stretch at 135 Degree to the Body:
- Hands Stretch Both Hands Straight Above the Head:
- Hands In and Out:

(C) Asanas (Yoga Postures)

Ardha Padmasana (Half Lotus Pose)

Procedure

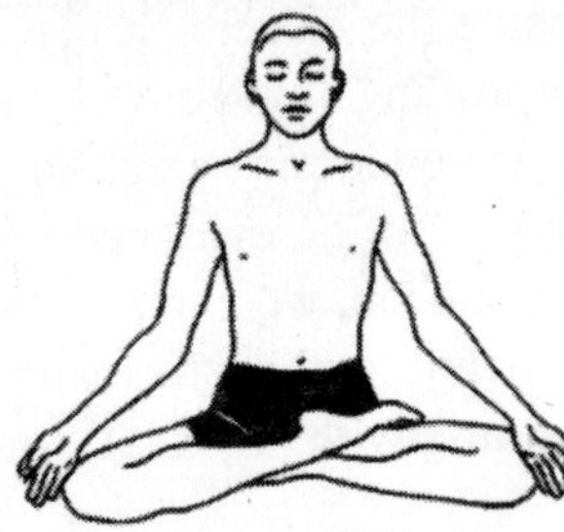

1. Sit with the legs straight in front of the body.
2. Bend one leg and place the sole of the foot on the inside of the opposite thigh. Bend the other leg and place the foot on top of the opposite thigh.
3. Without straining, try to place the upper heel as near as possible to the abdomen.
4. Adjust the position so that it is comfortable. Place the hands on the knees in *gyana mudra*. Keep the back, neck and head straight.

Benefits: Helps to practice in sitting for longer duration and keeps mind calm. It also helps to decrease muscular tension and blood pressure and also stimulates digestive process.

Ardha Ushtrasana (Half Camel Pose)

Procedure

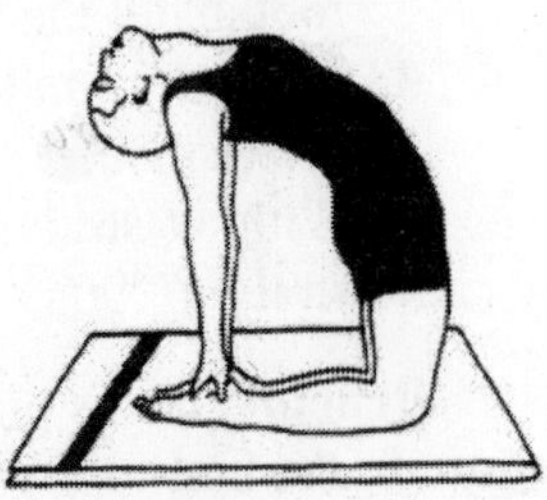

1. Sit in Vajrasana. Move the knees apart and the ankles to the side of the buttocks.
2. Stand up on the knees with the arms at the sides. Keep the feet flat behind the body. Stretch the arms sideways and raise them to shoulder level.
3. Twist to the right, reach back with the right hand and hold the right ankle.
4. Stretch the left arm, reach back and hold the left leg. The head should be slightly back with the eyes gazing at the upward. Push the hips forward in the final position and keep the thighs vertical.

Benefits: Improves the digestive and systems. Relieving backache and cures rounded back and drooping shoulders.

Makarasana (Crocodile Pose)

Procedure

1. Lie down on abdomen with legs spread out, toes remain out and heels inward.
2. Slowly fold the left hand at below the armpit. Place it on the right shoulder.
3. Likewise place the right arm on the left shoulder.
4. Place the head on the hands in a comfortable position.

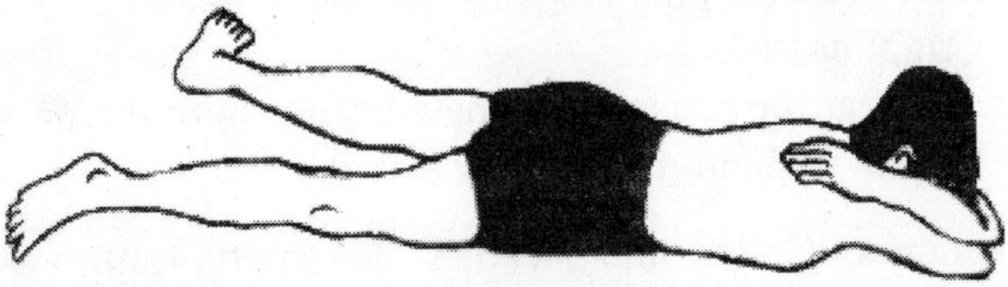

Benefits: Relaxes the whole body by relieving the physical and mental fatigue. Helps in relieving from back problems.

(D) Pranayama (Yoga Breathing Techniques)

Kapalbhati

Procedure

1. Sit in Padmasana, put both hands on respective knees. Exhale faster and forcibly through both the nostrils. Simultaneously draw the abdomen in.
2. After completing exhalation with force, take the breath in and bring the abdomen in previous position. The sound produced during inhalation and exhalation should be like a bellows of the blacksmith.

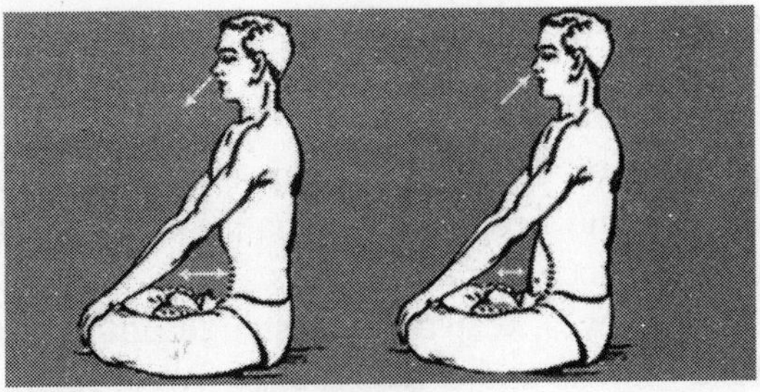

Benefits: Cleanses the naso-pharynx.

Anulom-Viloma (Alternate Nostril Breathing)

Procedure

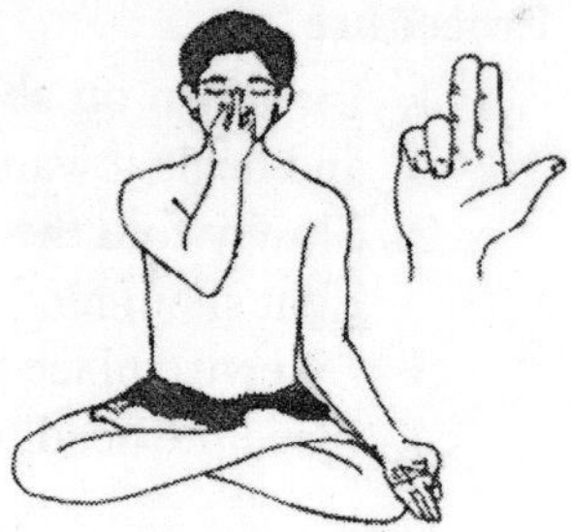

1. Sit in Padmasana with head and spine erect and eyes closed.
2. Close the right nostrils with the right thumb.
3. Inhale through the left nostril just before closing it with ring finger and release the air through the right nostril.
4. Repeat the process alternatively for both the nostrils about 5 times without making any sound.

Benefits: Calms and steadies the mind. Improves focus and concentration. Manages hypertension.

Bhramari (Bumble bee breathing)

Procedure

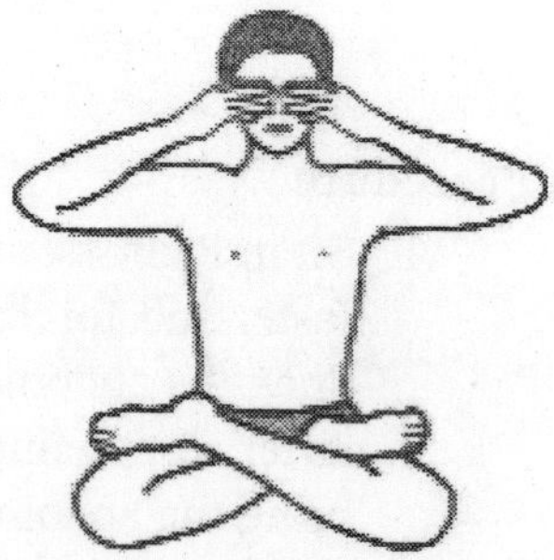

1. Sit in a comfortable meditative posture.
2. Using both the hands, place index finger on the forehead, close eyes with middle finger and close ears with thumbs with lips closed.
3. Inhale deeply and exhale by making a humming sound similar to black bee.

Benefits: Calms the mind and nervous system. Alleviates anger, anxiety and insomnia.

Guided Relaxation

1. Lie down on the ground. Keep a distance of one foot between the legs and keep both the hands open pointing upwards at some distance from the thighs.
2. Close the eyes, keep the neck straight and relax the whole body.
3. Gently inhale and exhale four to five deep breaths.

4. Now observe each part of the body through the mind with resolution and feeling that each part of the body is in a relaxed and stress-free state.
5. Do not sleep during the practice.

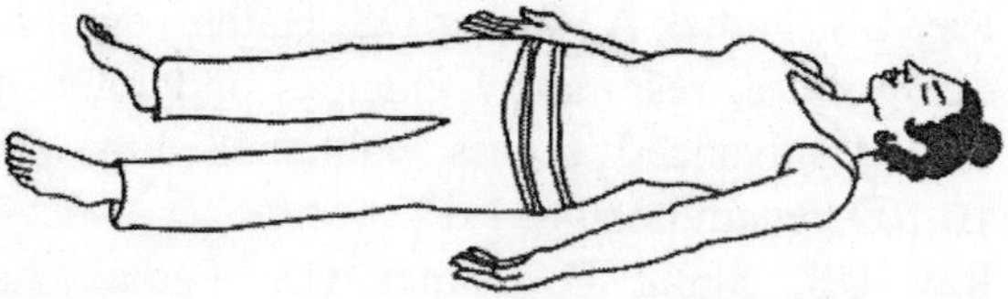

Benefits: Reduces mental stress, depression, high blood pressure, heart diseases and insomnia. The body, mind, brain and soul get complete rest, power, motivation and happiness. The concentration power is developed.

Acknowledgement: Authors are thankful to the Yoga group of DIPAS and Morarji Desai National Institute of Yoga for helpful discussions on different aspects of yogic asanas.

References

1. Joshi LN, Joshi VD, Gokhale LV. Effect of short term 'Pranayam' practice on breathing rate and ventilatory functions of lung. Indian J Physiol Pharmacol. 1992; 36(2):105-8.
2. Selvamurthy, W., Ray, U. S, Hegde, K. S & Sharma, R. P (1980) Physiological responses to cold (10 C) in men after six months practice of yogic practice. Int. J. Biometrol. 12, 188.
3. Himashree, G., Mohan, L., Singh, Y. Yoga Practice Improves Physiological and Biochemical Status at High Altitudes: A Prospective Case-control Study. Altern Ther Health Med. 2016;22(5):53-59.
4. Selvamurthy W, Ray US, Hedge KS and Sharma RP. Physiological responses to cold (10°C) in men after six months' practice of yoga exercises. Int J Biometeorol 1988; 32: 188 – 193.
5. Ray US, Hegde KS, Selvamurthy W. Effects of yogic asanas and physical exercises on body flexibility in middle – aged men. The Yoga Review 1983; 3: 75-79.
6. Ray US, Hegde KS, Selvamurthy W. Improvement in muscular efficiency as related to a standard task after yogic exercises in middle – aged men. Indian J. Med. Res 1986; 83: 343-348.

7. Ray US, Mukhopadhyaya S, Purkayastha SS, Asnani V, Tomer OS, Prashad R, Thakur L, Selvamurthy W. Effect of yogic exercises on physical and mental health of young fellowship course trainees. Indian J Physiol Pharmacol 2001a; 45:37-53.
8. Ray US, Pathak A, Tomer OS. Hatha yoga practices: Energy expenditure, respiratory changes and intensity of exercise. eCAM advanced access published June 21, 2010b. doi: 10.1093/ecam/neq046.1-12.
9. Ray US, Sinha B, Tomer OS, Pathak A, Dasgupta T, Selvamurthy W. Aerobic capacity & perceived exertion after practice of Hatha yogic exercises. Indian J Med Res 2001b; 114:215-221.
10. Pal R, Singh SN, Halder K, Tomer OS, Mishra AB, Saha M. Effect of yogic practices on age related changes in oxygen metabolism and antioxidant-redox status. J Exp Integr Med. 2013; 3(4): 305-312. doi:10.5455/jeim.060613.or.079.
11. Saha M, Halder K, Tomar OS, Pal R. Yoga: Environmental stress burster. *in Translational Research in Environmental and Occupational Stress. Springer India, 2014.*

8

Extreme Environment of Hot Deserts and Benefit from Yoga for Better Acclimatization

Heat is a natural hazard which drastically influences human health and well-being. As compared to other natural disasters, in many parts of the world, heat claims a greater number of lives. Yet, its gravity remains underestimated, since heat as a hazard suffers limited visibility. Hurricanes, floods and tornados are easily perceived, being more dramatic than heat waves (Schmeltz *et al.,* 2015).

In India, the summer months experience rising temperature and falling air pressure in the northern part of the country. A striking feature of the hot weather season is the 'loo'. These are strong, gusty, hot, dry winds blowing during the day over the north and northwestern India. Sometimes they even continue until late in the evening. Direct exposure to these winds may cause heat stress which could be fatal. In many occupations also heat stress is an issue all year round (such as bakeries, compressed air tunnels, foundries and smelting operations), where there may be an increased risk of heat stress for some people. Heat stress occurs when the body's means of controlling its internal temperature starts to fail.

The spectrum of heat related illnesses (HRIs) ranges from relatively mild heat exhaustion and cramps to the deleterious, life-threatening heat stroke. Severe HRI, in clinical terms, can be described as a blend of cytotoxicity and systematic inflammatory response, which may result in multiple organ failure, if left untreated (Li *et al.,* 2014). With rise in global temperature, HRIs are continue to increase in severity worldwide. The identification and estimation of heat-related morbidity and mortality is a major challenge. Heat stress manifests itself into respiratory, cardiovascular, and cerebrovascular disorders, leading to the attribution of the deaths caused by heat stress to these disorders (Schmeltz *et al.,* 2015; Atha, 2013; Santelli *et al.,* 2014; Donoghue *et al.,* 1997; Rogers *et al.,* 2007; Jay *et al.,* 2010).

The distinction between the diagnosis of heat exhaustion and heatstroke is perplexing, since these conditions are defined based on a range of core body temperatures (CBT), and symptoms that are similar and sizeably overlapping. Due to the blurred lines and lack of definite markers, the decision of hospitalizing the patient (under mild heat stress) or otherwise (under severe heat stress) is based solely on the discretion of the physician.

Human studies on physiology of exercise in hyperthermia, albeit successful in providing important information, suffer with basic limitation that they can only reveal partial information regarding the pathophysiology of the life-threatening heat stroke (King *et al.,* 2015).

Various cooling methods, for management of heat stroke have been investigated. The most effective method is considered to be cold water emersion followed by conductive cooling. These methods most efficiently reduced body temperature. When the feasibility of ice-water immersion is less, continual wetting with water coupled with patient fanning is adopted. There is a threat of patients becoming hypothermic upon such aggressive cooling. Keeping this limitation in view, 38.6°C is considered a limit to the degree of active cooling (King *et al.,* 2015; McDermott *et al.,* 2009; Demartini *et al.,* 2015; Flouris *et al.,* 2015; Lee *et al.,* 2012). Additionally, HRIs are associated with a wide array of physiological responses that vary between individuals. There is response variability, both at the time of heat stress and subsequent recovery. In addition to this, the extremely complex etiology of heat stress, makes severity testing extremely challenging.

Thermoregulation in Human

Hypothalamus is the thermoregulatory centre which controls the body temperature in humans. It receives input from two sets of thermoreceptors:

Receptors in the hypothalamus itself monitor the temperature of the blood as it passes through the brain (the core temperature), and receptors in the skin monitor the external temperature. Both sets of information are needed so that the body can make appropriate adjustments. The thermoregulatory centre sends impulses to several different effectors to adjust body temperature:

The first response to encountering hotter or colder condition is voluntary — if too hot, we may decide to take some clothes off, or to move into the shade; if too cold, we put extra clothes on — or turn the heating up! It is only when these responses are not enough that the thermoregulatory centre is stimulated. This is part of the autonomic nervous system, so the various responses are all involuntary. When we get too hot, the heat loss centre in the hypothalamus is stimulated; when we get too cold, it is the heat conservation centre of the hypothalamus which is stimulated. Note that some of the responses to low temperature actually generate heat (thermogenesis), whilst others just conserve heat. Similarly some of the responses to heat actively cool the body down, while others just reduce heat production or transfer heat to the surface. The body thus has a range of responses available, depending on the internal and external temperatures.

Epidemiology of Heat Exposure

Heat stress is one of those environmental stresses to which almost every individual is exposed, at some time or the other during his/her lifetime (Leithead and Lind., 1964). It was earlier believed that human beings could inhabit and thrive under any temperature conditions, no matter how high the temperature, since already, most of the hot regions on earth are inhabited. Sherwood and Huber contradicted this view and proved that there is a limit to the 'peak heat stress value', beyond which adaptation is not possible (Sherwood and Huber, 2010). The global average temperature, by the end of this century, has been predicted to increase by 1.8°C – 4.0°C (IPCC, 2007).

There are estimates suggesting that doubling of CO_2 concentration corresponds with1.9°C – 4.5°C rise in global temperature. There is a projection through conclusions of different studies that by the year 2300, the combustion of fossil fuels will result in a rise in CO_2 concentration by 2.75 fold, which would further increase global temperature by 12 °C. As global temperatures increase by 7°C, small zones will be created, where metabolic heat will not be dissipated and there will be a more severe increase of 11–12 °C, leading to the expansion of the zones to cover all the inhabited areas on earth (Donoghue *et al.,* 1997).

Also, there is a very high probability of increase in the frequency of extreme heat events such as deleterious heat waves resulting in an increased risk of HRIs induced morbidity and mortality (Meehl and Tebaldi, 2004; Vandentorren *et al.,* 2004).

Deaths rate was found to be 688 persons per year based on the recordings of average annual death/year over 5 years out of 3,442 total deaths in USA due to HRIs (Luber and McGeehin, 2008). About 423 heat-related deaths were observed among crop workers in USA from 1992 to 2006 (Kjellstrom, 2009; MMWR, 2008). In France, more than 50 years record was broken during the 2003 European heat wave with temperatures exceeding those of previously observed heat waves (1976, 1983, and 1994) (Vandentorren *et al.,* 2004). In 2003, 1,065 people died of acute heat wave in the southern Indian state of Andhra Pradesh (BBC, 2012). Apart from these deaths due to classical form of HRI, the mortality due to exertional HRI is also prevalent. Soldiers, athletes, farmers, miners etc. perform strenuous physical activity for extended durations in hot weather producing high levels of metabolic heat, rendering them susceptible to HRIs (Wyndham, 1967; Carter *et al.,* 2005; Mirabelli *et al.,* 2010; Jackson and Rosenberg, 2010). Malholtra and Venkataswamy reported that about 90 % of the total heat causalities in military personnel occurred in recruits in various military training centres and remaining 10% were seen amongst the trained soldiers (Malholtra and Venkataswamy, 1974). Local climatic changes are likely to create occupational health risks and significantly affect the productivity of the employees, hampering the socio-economic environment of the affected countries in the long run (Kjellstrom, 2009). Heat-related deaths at work have occasionally been reported, the first report is on the outcomes of the classical studies in South Africa (Wyndham, 1965). Alzeer *et al.,* 1997 reported that about 2 million people perform pilgrimage to Mecca every year. Mecca lies at a latitude of 20°N and the temperature exceeds 45°C during summer. Lack of acclimatization and physical exertion render these pilgrims susceptible to heat stroke (Alzeer *et al.,* 1997).

Despite of HRIs being preventable (Becker and Stewart, 2011; Lee-Chiong and Stitt, 1995; Sandor, 1997; MMWR, 1995) heat stroke remains the third leading cause of mortality in US high school athletes (Barrow and Clark; 1998). The mortality because of HRIs is under-reported as deaths mostly occur due to respiratory, cardiovascular and cerebrovascular disorders during heat waves and strenuous physical activity in hot climate (Barrow and Clark; 1998). Physiological and behavioural adaptations may reduce morbidity and mortality due to HRIs (McGeehin and Mirabelli, 2001). In depth research in this field is required so that certain adverse health effects can be avoided, prevented and treated as required.

Heat-Related Illness: An Overview

Types of HRIs

HRIs cover an entire spectrum, from minor to life threatening, including i) heat stress/cramps, ii) heat exhaustion (relatively milder) and iii) heatstroke (life threatening).

i) Heat Cramps

Heat Cramps are a milder form of HRIs, observed in both un-acclimated individuals (at the beginning of strenuous physical activity in hot temperatures) and heat-acclimatized individuals, who have been sweating profusely while physical activity, if, in particular, rehydrating with unsalted fluids such as plain water. The cramps usually affect exercising muscle groups but may affect any other muscle as well. The cramping may occur both during the activity or hours later. Cramping may be caused if the fluid losses are compensated with hypotonic solutions (Eichner, 2007).

ii) Heat Exhaustion

Heat exhaustion is a clinical condition associated with headache, vomiting, nausea, lethargy, and thirst (Ahmed *et al.,* 1996; Costrini *et al.,* 1979). Exposure to elevated temperatures, sweating, and failure of proper replenishment of salt and water are the underlying factors. Broadly, heat exhaustion is of two types-

Exposure to high temperature coupled with insufficient fluid intake result in water depletion heat exhaustion with symptom onset manifesting over a few hours. On the contrary, the salt depletion subtype of heat exhaustion usually manifests over several days; generally in individuals that though replace fluid loses adequately, fail at replacing salt loses. The symptoms include thirst, nausea, headache and vomiting. The associated temperature range is from normal to elevated, usually <40 degrees. Tachycardia and tachypnea are observed. Impending heatstroke and shocks are the associated complications. In most cases, patients tend to experience both types of heat exhaustion in combination (Louie, 2009).

iii) Heatstroke

It is a life threatening physiological state characterized by CBT > 40 degrees, associated neurological dysfunction, and absence of sweating. Heatstroke is observed when the body fails to dissipate heat resulting in malfunctioning temperature control. This drastic rise in CBT results in cellular and organ level injuries. The associated metabolic abnormalities include renal failure, hepatocellular necrosis, rhabdomyolysis, cerebral edema, myocardial damage, and metabolic abnormalities of various types. There are associated hyperventilation and tachycardia under heat stroke, along with respiratory alkalosis and metabolic acidosis.

Heatstroke can be divided into 2 subtypes;

a. Classic or Non-exertional heatstroke

This subtype is commonly seen in elderly, infants, and children. It takes a few days to develop, usually during a heat wave and presents with vomiting, nausea, headache, and a worsening mental status.

b. Exertional heatstroke

It is usually seen in young, exercising individuals who are not heat acclimatised. Central nervous system changes are observed, that range from severe headache to collapse and seizures. Disseminated intravascular coagulation (DIC) and rhabdomyolysis are prominent. Severe lactic acidosis also develops during early onset but it is not a prognostic indicator for classic heatstroke (U.S. Department of health and human services, https://chemm.nlm.nih.gov/heatstress.htm; Tokizawa *et al.,* 2015; Hubbard, 1990; Chung and Pin, 1996; Howe and Boden, 2007; Crider *et al.,* 2014).

Yoga Helps for Better Acclimatization in Hot Desert Condition

One of the extreme climatic environmental conditions that exist on earth is the desert where temperature reaches more than 55°C in daytime and subzero in night time with 10% humidity and minimum rainfall. The terrain condition is always dry in nature with sand or dust storm, solar radiation and disturbed working schedule. These critical factors are responsible for disturbing body's homeostasis, hyperthermia, heatstroke, dryness in skin, feeling thirsty always, and frequent feeling of fatigue without much workout. Prevention of water loss by breathing through nostrils instead of breathing through mouth may be beneficial in such weather conditions. One should avoid smoking at desert conditions while plenty of water should be taken to counter dehydration. Working under direct sun should be avoided.

As a counter measure, to get rid of these conditions, practice of specific yogic breathing exercise and asana shall be beneficial. Practicing of cooling pranayama like Sheetkari, Sheetali may be helpful for maintaining proper body homeostasis as well as cooling down the body in hot environment. Vigorous energy consuming exercises should be avoided to prevent excessive water loss through sweating. Work may be advised to be done under shed with fully covered clothing. Thus, Yoga can serve as a very good alternative in these circumstances as the energy expenditure of the asana, pranayama is very less than conventional exercises (Samantha et al, 2013).

Special Yoga Package for Comabating Heat Stress:

(A) Universal Prayer

(B) Guided Relaxation

Procedure

1. Lie down on the ground. Keep a distance of one foot between the legs and keep both the hands open pointing upwards at some distance from the thighs.
2. Close the eyes, keep the neck straight and relax the whole body. Gently inhale and exhale four to five deep breaths.
3. Now observe each part of the body through the mind with resolution and feeling that each part of the body is in a relaxed and stress-free state.
4. Do not sleep during the practice.

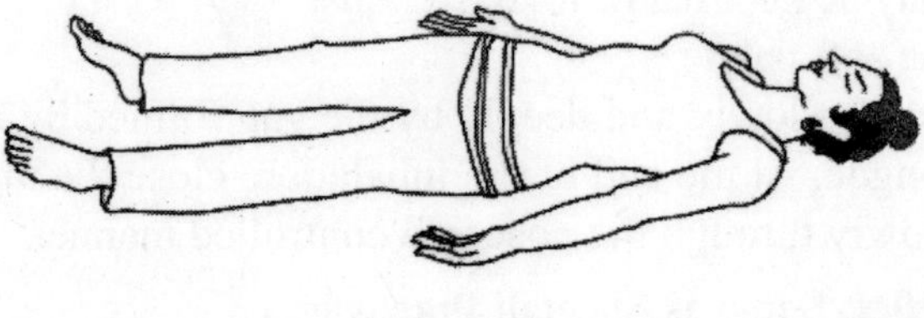

Benefits: Reduces mental stress, depression, high blood pressure, heart diseases and insomnia. The body, mind, brain and soul get complete rest, power, motivation and happiness. The concentration power is developed.

(C) Pranayama (Yoga Breathing Techniques)

Cooling Pranayama: Sheetali

Procedure

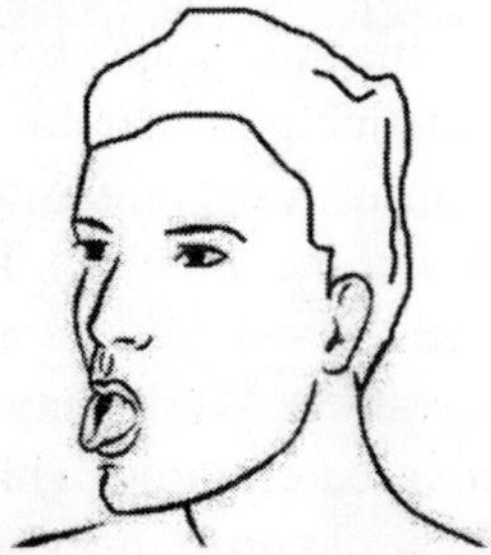

1. Sit in any comfortable meditation posture. Close the eyes and relax the whole body.
2. Extend the tongue outside the mouth as far as possible without strain. Roll the sides of the tongue up so that it forms a tube.
3. Slowly inhale through the rolled tongue. At the end of inhalation, draw the tongue in, close the mouth and exhale through the nose.

Benefits: This practice cools the body and affects important brain centres associated with biological drives and temperature regulation. It cools and reduces mental and emotional excitation. It induces muscular relaxation and mental tranquillity.

(D) Sitkari

Procedure

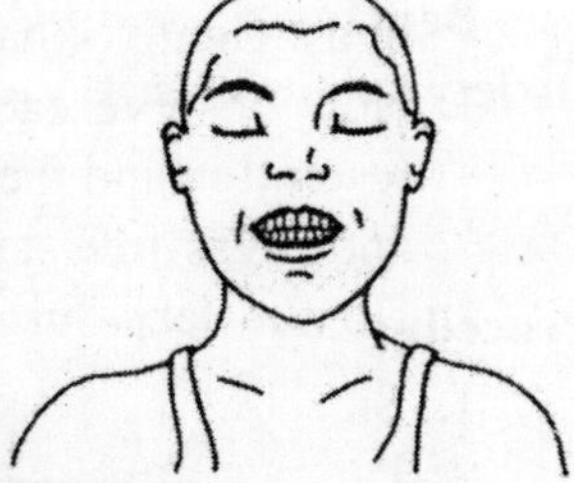

1. Sit in any comfortable meditation posture. Close the eyes and relax the whole body. Hold the teeth lightly together. Separate the lips, exposing the teeth. The tongue may be kept flat or folded against the soft palate.
2. Inhale slowly and deeply by the gap formed by both sides of tongue. At the end of the inhalation, close the mouth. Exhale slowly through the nose in a controlled manner.

Benefits: Same as Sheetali Pranayama.

Sadanta

Procedure

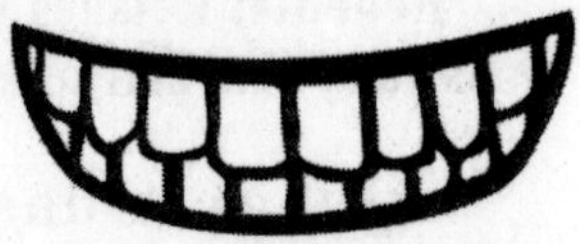

1. Sit in any comfortable meditation posture. Close the eyes and relax the whole body.
2. Let the upper teeth touches the lower teeth. Separate the lips, exposing the teeth.
3. The tip of the tongue touches the teeth.
4. Inhale through the crevices of the teeth and the air moves over the gums slowly and continuously into the mouth and passes down the trachea into the lungs.
5. Exhale slowly through the nose in a controlled manner.

Benefits: Same as Sheetali Pranayama.

Bhramari Pranayama

Procedure

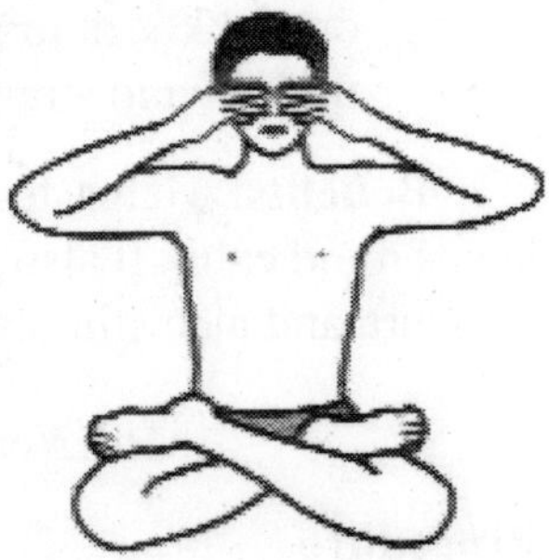

1. Sit in the position of Padmasana.
2. Using both the hands, place index finger on the forehead, close eyes with middle finger and close ears with the thumbs with lips closed.
3. Inhale deeply and exhale by making a humming sound similar to black bee.

Benefits: Clams the mind and nervous system. Allevates anger, anxiety and insomnia.

Meditative Breathing

Procedure

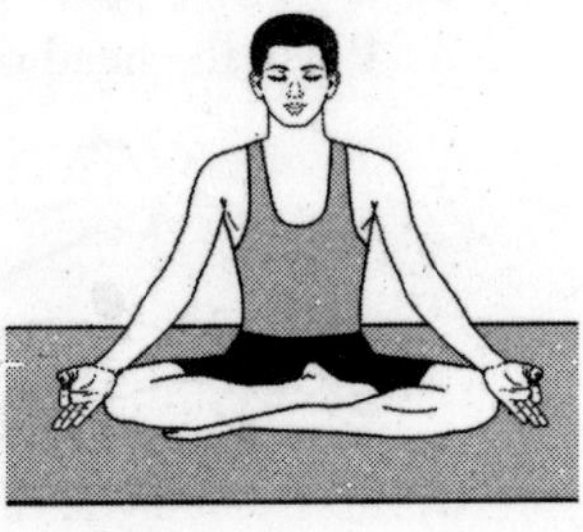

1. Sit in a meditative posture Padmasana. Breathe through both nostrils with closed eyes.
2. Observe your breath and feel air is passing from nose, trachea and lung.

3. At last blink the eyes slowly and come out of mediation.

Benefits: Relaxes whole body and mind reduces blood pressure, respiratory rate and stress. Gives feeling of complete well-being.

Asanas: Ardha Padmasana (Half Lotus Pose)

Procedure

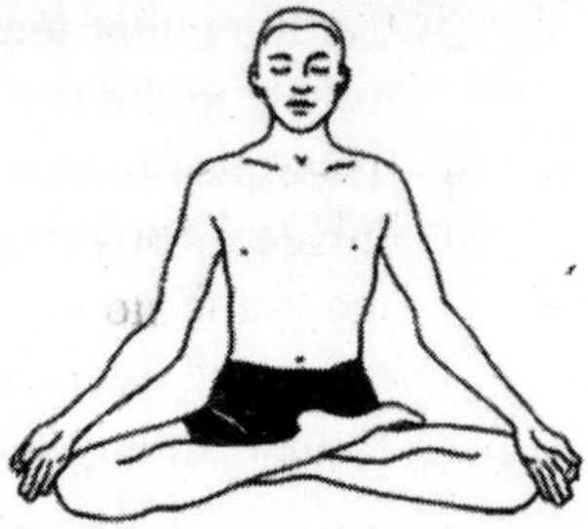

1. Sit with the legs straight in front of the body.
2. Bend one leg and place the sole of the foot on the inside of the opposite thigh. Bend the other leg and place the foot on top of the opposite thigh.
3. Without straining, try to place the upper heel as near as possible to the abdomen.
4. Adjust the position so that it is comfortable. Place the hands on the knees in gyana mudra. Keep the back, neck and head upright and straight.

Benefits: Helps to practice of sitting for longer duration and keeps mind calm. It also helps to decrease muscular tension and blood pressure and also stimulates digestive process.

Makarasana (Crocodile Pose)

Procedure

1. Lie down on abdomen with legs spread out, toes remain out and heels inward.
2. Slowly fold the left hand at below the armpit. Place it on the right shoulder.
3. Likewise place the right arm on the left shoulder.
4. Place the head on the hands in a comfortable position.

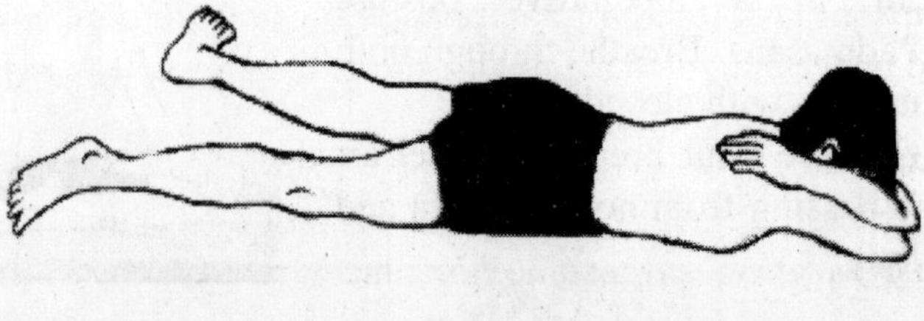

Benefits: Relaxes the whole body by relieving the physical and mental fatigue. Helps in relieving from back problems.

Shavasana (Corpse Pose)

Procedure

1. Lie down on back and place hands near the thighs and palm facing upwards.
2. Keep the heels slightly apart and toes pointing outwards with relaxed body.

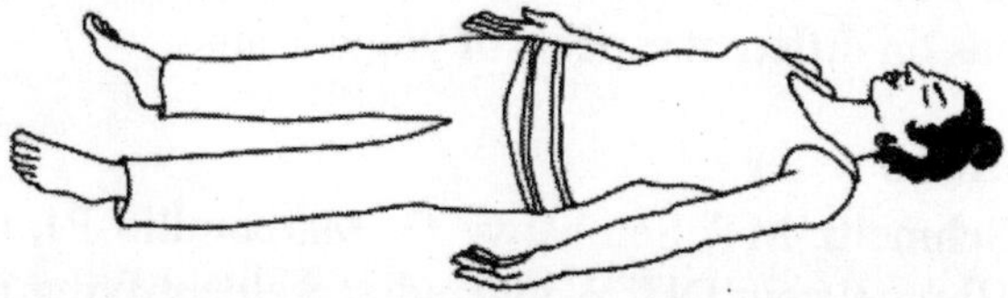

Benefits: Relaxes whole body. Relieves physical and mental fatigue. Extremely beneficial for high blood pressure.

Sukhasana

Procedure

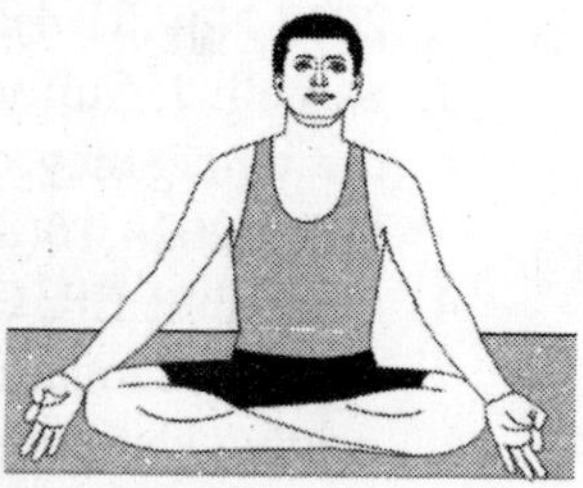

1. Sit with the legs straight in front of the body.
2. Bend one leg and place the foot under the opposite thigh.
3. Bend the other leg and place the foot under the opposite thigh.
4. Place the hands on the knees in gyana mudra.
5. Without straining keep the head, neck and back upright and straight. Relax the whole body.

Benefits: Brings mental and physical balance without causing any strain in the body.

Caution: All the yogic practices described here should be practiced under the guidance of an experienced Yoga teacher.

Conclusion

In general, regular yogic practices help to achieve a better autonomic balance, orthostatic tolerance, relative hypo-metabolic state, and thermoregulatory efficiency to heat stress. It also gives benefits to the practitioners with increased vitality, improved lung functions, delineated psychological stress, reduced cardiovascular stress and improved antioxidant and redox status. A combination of yogic asanas, pranayamas and meditation are beneficial for the combatants working in hot and tropical conditions to cope up with the adverse climate along with the execution of regular assigned duties as well as for mental well-being.

Acknowledgement: Authors are thankful to the Yoga group of DIPAS and Morarji Desai National Institute of Yoga for helpful discussions on different aspects of yogic asanas.

References

1. Schmeltz MT, Sembajwe G, Marcotullio PJ, Grassman JA, Himmelstein DU, Woolhandler S. Identifying individual risk factors and documenting the pattern of heat-related illness through analyses of hospitalization and patterns of household cooling. PLoS One. 2015;10(3):e0118958.
2. Atha WF. Heat-related illness. Emerg Med Clin North Am. 2013 Nov;31(4):1097-108
3. Santelli J, Sullivan JM, Czarnik A, Bedolla J. Heat illness in the emergency department: keeping your cool. Emerg Med Pract. 2014;16(8):1-21; quiz 21-2.
4. Donoghue ER, Graham MA, Jentzen JM, Lifschultz BD, Luke JL, Mirchandani HG. Criteria for the diagnosis of heat-related deaths: National Association of Medical Examiners. Position paper. National Association of Medical Examiners Ad Hoc Committee on the Definition of Heat-Related Fatalities. Am J Forensic Med Pathol. 1997;18(1):11-4.
5. Rogers B, Stiehl K, Borst J, Hess A, Hutchins S. Heat-related illnesses: the role of the occupational and environmental health nurse. AAOHN J. 2007;55(7):279-87; quiz 288-9.
6. Jay O, Kenny GP. Heat exposure in the Canadian workplace. Am J Ind Med. 2010;53(8):842-53.
7. King MA, Leon LR, Mustico DL, Haines JM, Clanton TL. Biomarkers of multiorgan injury in a preclinical model of exertional heat stroke. J Appl Physiol (1985). 2015;118(10):1207-20.

8. McDermott BP, Casa DJ, O'Connor FG, Adams WB, Armstrong LE, Brennan AH, Lopez RM, Stearns RL, Troyanos C, Yeargin SW. Cold-water dousing with ice massage to treat exertional heat stroke: a case series. Aviat Space Environ Med. 2009;80(8):720-2.
9. Demartini JK, Casa DJ, Stearns R, Belval L, Crago A, Davis R, Jardine J. Effectiveness of cold water immersion in the treatment of exertional heat stroke at the Falmouth Road Race. Med Sci Sports Exercise. 2015; 47(2):240-5.
10. Flouris AD, Friesen BJ, Carlson MJ, Casa DJ, Kenny GP. Effectiveness of cold water immersion for treating exertional heat stress when immediate response is not possible. Scand J Med Sci Sports. 2015;25 Suppl 1:229-39.
11. Lee EC, Watson G, Casa D, Armstrong LE, Kraemer W, Vingren JL, Spiering BA, Maresh CM. Interleukin-6 responses to water immersion therapy after acute exercise heat stress: a pilot investigation. J Athl Train. 2012 Nov-Dec;47(6):655-63.
12. Sherwood SC, Huber M. An adaptability limit to climate change due to heat stress. Proc Natl Acad Sci U S A. 2010;107(21):9552-5.
13. IPCC, 2007: Climate Change 2007: Impacts, Adaptation and Vulnerability. Contribution of Working Group II to the Fourth Assessment Report of the Intergovernmental Panel on Climate Change, M.L. Parry, O.F. Canziani, J.P. Palutikof, P.J. van der Linden and C.E. Hanson, Eds., Cambridge University Press, Cambridge, UK, 976pp.
14. Meehl GA, Tebaldi C. More intense, more frequent, and longer lasting heat waves in the 21st century. Science. 2004; 305(5686):994-7.
15. Vandentorren S, Suzan F, Medina S, Pascal M, Maulpoix A, Cohen JC, Ledrans M. Mortality in 13 French cities during the August 2003 heat wave. Am J Public Health. 2004; 94(9):1518-20.
16. Luber G, McGeehin M. Climate change and extreme heat events. Am J Prev Med. 2008; 35(5):429-35.
17. Kjellstrom T. Climate change, direct heat exposure, health and well-being in low and middle-income countries. Glob Health Action. 2009; 2.

18. Heat-related deaths among crop workers- United States, 1992-2006. MMWR. JAMA 2008; 300:1017-8.
19. British Broadcasting Corporation India. Heat deaths exceed 1,000. Available at: http://news.bbc.co.uk/2/hi/south_asia/2956490.stm. Accessed 8 Oct 2012.
20. Wyndham C, Benade A, Williams C, Strydom N, Goldin A, Heyns A. Changes in central circulation and body fluid spaces during acclimatization to heat. J Appl Physiol 1968; 25: 586–593.
21. Carter R 3rd, Cheuvront S, Williams J, Kolka M, Stephenson L, Sawka M et al. Epidemiology of hospitalizations and deaths from heat illness in soldiers. Med Sci Sports Exerc 2005;37:1338-1344.
22. Mirabelli MC, Quandt SA, Crain R, Grzywacz JG, Robinson EN, Vallejos QM, Arcury TA. Symptoms of heat illness among Latino farm workers in North Carolina. American Journal of Preventive Medicine. 2010; 39(5), 468-471.
23. Jackson LL, Rosenberg HR. Preventing heat-related illness among agricultural workers. Journal of Agromedicine. 2010;15(3),200-215.
24. Malhotra MS and venkataswamy Y. Heat casualty in the Indian armed forces. Indian Journal of Medical Research.1974; 62, 1293-1302.
25. Wyndham C. A survey of the causal factors in heat stroke and of their prevention in the gold mining industry. J S African Inst Mining and Metallurg 1965;66: 125-55.
26. Alzeer AH, el-Hazmi MA, Warsy AS, Ansari ZA, Yrkendi MS. Serum enzymes in heat stroke: prognostic implication. Clin Chem. 1997;43(7):1182-7.
27. Becker J, Stewart L. Heat-related illness. AmFam Physician 2011; 83:1325-1330.
28. Lee-Chiong T Jr, Stitt J. Heatstroke and other heat-related illnesses. The maladies of summer. Postgrad Med 1995; 98:26–36.
29. Sandor R. Heat illness: on site diagnosis and cooling. Physician Sportsmed 1997; 25:35–40.
30. Heat-related illness and deaths—United States, 1994–1995 MMWR Morb Mortal Wkly Rep 1995; 44:465–468.

31. Barrow M, Clark K. Heat-related illnesses. Am Fam Physician 1998; 58:749-756.
32. McGeehin M, Mirabelli M. The potential impacts of climate variability and change on temperature-related morbidity and mortality in the United States. Environ Health Prospect 2001; 109 Suppl 2:185-189.
33. Eichner ER. The role of sodium in 'heat cramping'. Sports Med.2007;37(4-5):368-70.
34. Ahmed A, Sadaniantz A. Metabolic and electrolyte abnormalities during heat exhaustion. Postgrad Med J. 1996;72(850):505-6.
35. Costrini AM, Pitt HA, Gustafson AB, Uddin DE. Cardiovascular and metabolic manifestations of heat stroke and severe heat exhaustion. Am J Med. 1979;66(2):296-302.
36. Louie RF, Sumner SL, Belcher S, Mathew R, Tran NK, Kost GJ. Thermal stress and point-of-care testing performance: suitability of glucose test strips and bloodgas cartridges for disaster response. Disaster Med Public Health Prep. 2009;3(1):13-7.
37. Tokizawa K, Sawada S, Tai T, Lu J, Oka T, Yasuda A, Takahashi M. Effects of partial sleep restriction and subsequent daytime napping on prolonged exertional heat strain. Occup Environ Med. 2015; 72(7):521-8.
38. Hubbard RW. Heatstroke pathophysiology: the energy depletion model. Med Sci Sports Exercise 1990;22(1):19-28.
39. Chung NK, Pin CH. Obesity and the occurrence of heat disorders. Mil Med. 1996;161(12):739-42.
40. Howe AS, Boden BP. Heat-related illness in athletes. Am J Sports Med. 2007; 35(8):1384-95.
41. Crider KG, Maples EH, Gohlke JM. Incorporating occupational risk in heat stress vulnerability mapping. J Environ Health. 2014; 77(1):16-22.
42. Samantha W, Jayasinghe MTR, Goswami YD. Identifying the adaptive opportunities in factory environments for a better thermal comfort-preliminary studies. 2013.

❐

9
Confined Environment of Submarine and Yoga

The environment in a submarine is one where human being faces physical and psychological limitations. A deep understanding of human physiology and adaptability is needed to ensure safety and efficiency of human operations underwater. Submarines, unlike surface ships, by virtue of the medium that they operate in, are susceptible to a distinct set of problems which are quite different from those experienced by surface ships. Any disaster in a submarine at depth needs a well-trained and efficient team, geared up to meet various contingencies that are bound to come up. This would be essential to prevent/reduce morbidity and mortality normally associated with such events.

Submarine personnel are exposed to extreme environmental challenges. At any given time, submariners are sealed in tiny living spaces, exposed to manufactured air and artificial light, and submerged to great depths for an excess of days. During this time, their job is to operate an extremely complicated and potentially dangerous machine. Their confinement in this small, artificial ecological unit leads to changes in their physiology. Submariners are exposed to gases which may lead to enhance stressful conditions. Another important aspect of the submarine environment is the prolonged isolation. This imposed isolation can involve 60 to 90 days of submerged cruising, and researchers have found several problems may arise such as fatigue, muscular tension, low motivation, disruption of circadian cycles, and minor emotional disturbances (Tansey *et al.,* 1979; Sosiukin *et al.,* 2014;). The submarine environment's effect on cardiovascular health has been considered in a number of studies. Findings showed that, as a direct result of limited exercise space, the physical activity level is low; however, weight gain by the crew was minimal and did not present a problem (Beare *et al.,* 1981). Other submarine environment-related problems include a lack of appropriate environmental cues being implicated in circadian cycle disintegration and a decrement in sleep quality. The confining nature of the submarine, with its constant requirement for optical accommodation and convergence was related to visual deteriorations.

DRDO has established a hyperbaric chamber at INS Aswani which is used for the treatment of decompression illnesses. These chambers are specific for treatment of diving and submarine accidents besides a variety of medical and surgical diseases. Hyperbaric oxygen therapy is very effective for the successful treatment of burns, crush injuries, gangrene etc.

During submarine escape or diving operations arterial gas embolism may occur which is a potentially catastrophic event that occurs when gas bubbles enter or form in the arterial vasculature and block it, causing organ ischemia. Surgeon Rear Admiral MS Malhotra along with HC Wright published a paper in 1961where they reported that the rabbits were exposed to a simulated depth of 100 ft. of water in a pressure chamber, and then during decompression, the trachea was closed at a 'depth of 60 ft.' until the surface was reached. Under these conditions the main injuries observed in a series of 10 experimental animals were, air embolism, pneumothorax and interstitial emphysema. In those cases where pneumothorax was present, the quantity of air in the blood vessels was small or absent altogether. Air appeared in the circulation only after the intra-tracheal pressure was allowed to return to atmospheric. Manual squeezing of the chest or applying an abdominal binder prior to clamping the trachea were both found to be effective in preventing these injuries in a further series of 10 rabbits. Squeezing the chest reduces the volume of air in the lungs to nearly residual. The binder not only reduces the initial lung volume by raising the diaphragm, but also provides support to the lungs during decompression. In a few human trials, subjects ascending from a depth of 100 ft. found the ascent to be more comfortable when wearing an abdominal binder than without one (Malhotra and Wright, 1961).

The Defence Institute of Physiology and Allied Sciences (DIPAS), one of DRDO's life sciences laboratories, has developed a customised yoga package to submarine soldiers. Yoga (asana and pranayama) are beneficial for improving soldiers' mental and physical condition in a submarine environment. For submariners, there are space constraints; hence exercises are performed in sitting or standing posture, yoga helps in better cognition and sleep.

Yoga module for Submarine
Universal Prayer
Loosening Exercises

Surya Namaskar (Sun Salutation)

Position I: Pranamasana

Procedure

1. Stand with the feet together and arms by the sides.
2. Keep the eyes closed.
3. Slowly bend the elbows and place together in front of the chest in Namaskara mudra and relax the whole body.

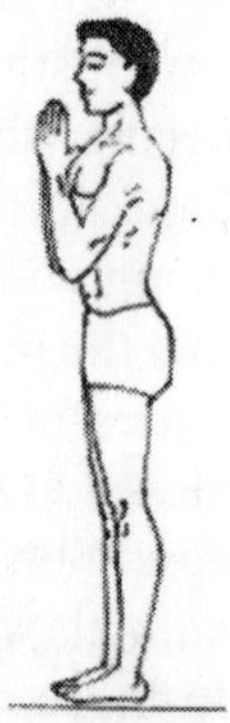

Benefits: Increases concentration and calmness.

Position II: Hasta Utthanasana

Procedure

1. Separate the hands, raise and stretch both arms above the head, keeping them shoulder width apart.
2. Bend the head, arms and upper trunk slightly backward.

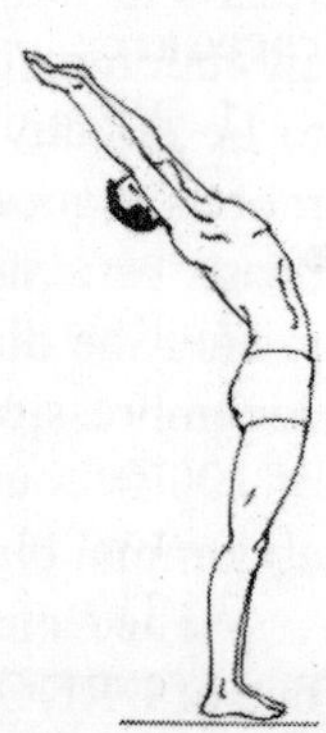

Benefits: Improves digestion and lung capacity.

Position III: Padahastasana

Procedure

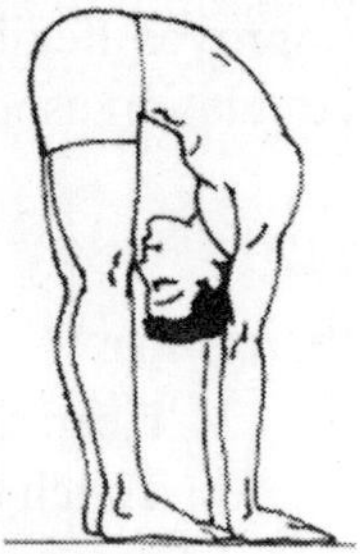

1. Bend forward from the hips until the fingers or palms of the hands touch the floor on either side of the feet.
2. Keep the knees straight and bring the forehead as close as possible to the knee.

Benefits: Improves digestion, removes flatulence and indigestion.

Position IV: Ashwa Sanchalanasana

Procedure

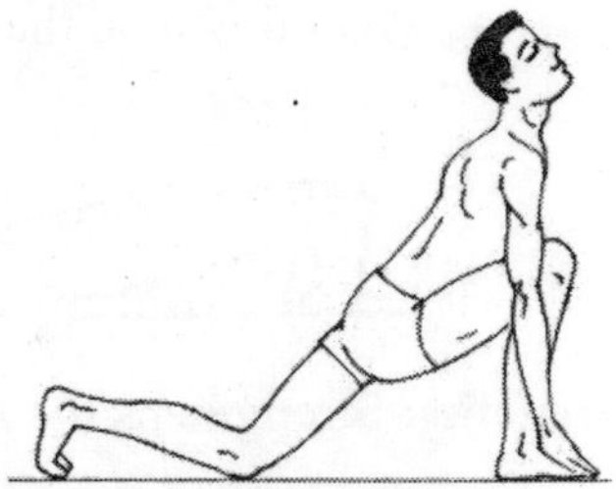

1. Place the hands on the floor beside the feet. Stretch the right leg as far as comfortable and grasp the floor with the toes.
2. Bend the left knee, keeping the left foot on the floor in the same position. Keep the arms straight.
3. The head should be tilted backward. The back arched and the inner gaze directed upward to the eyebrow centre.

Benefits: Tones abdominal organs. Strengthens arm, feet, ankle, legs and hips.

Position V: Parvatasana

Procedure

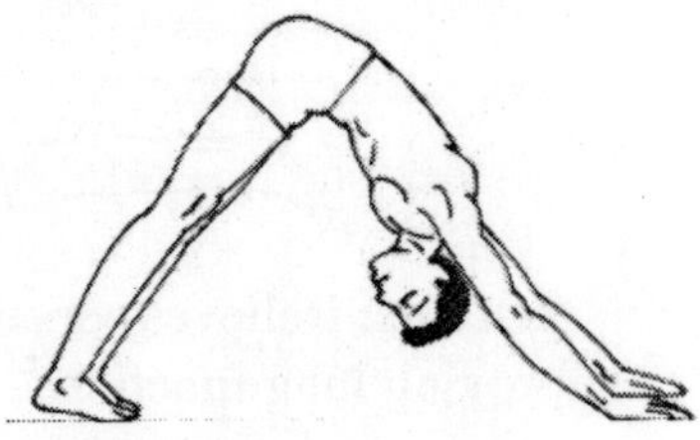

1. Keep the hands and right foot still and take the left foot back besides the right foot.
2. Raise the buttocks and lower the head between the arms so that the back and legs form two sides of a triangle.
3. The legs and arms straighten in the final position and the heels come down towards the floor in the final pose.

4. Bring the head and shoulders towards the knees.

Benefits: Strengthens the muscles and nerves in the back and legs. Improves flexibility by stretching muscles and ligaments. Improves circulation especially in the upper spine between shoulder blades.

Position VI: Astanga Namaskara

Procedure

1. Keep the hands and feet in place.
2. Touch the knees, chest and chin to the floor, the feet will come up on to the toes.
3. In the final position only the toes, knees, chest, hands and chin touch the floor.
4. Press down on the arm.

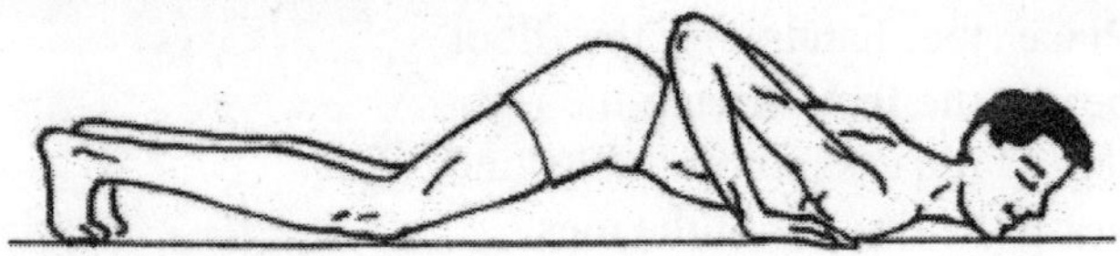

Benefits: Strengthens the arms, shoulder and leg muscle.

Position VII: Bhujangasana

Procedure

1. Lie down on abdomen with legs close together to the ground.
2. Place hands besides the body with palm touching on ground.
3. Lift the prone body from the ground up to the naval region.

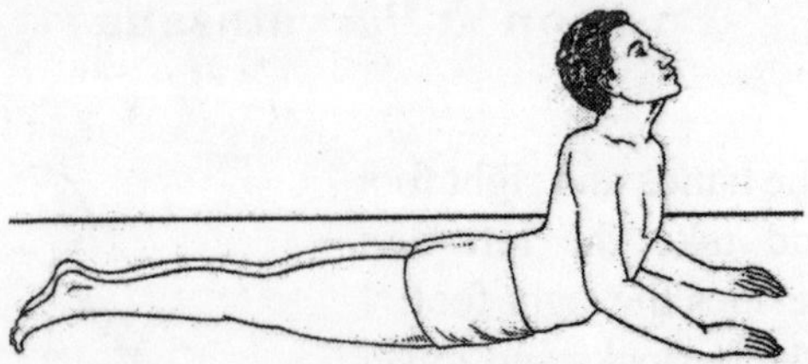

Benefits: Relieves constipation, indigestion and flatulence. Helps in improving lung function.

Position VIII: Parvatasana

Procedure: Same as position-V.

Benefits: Same as position-V.

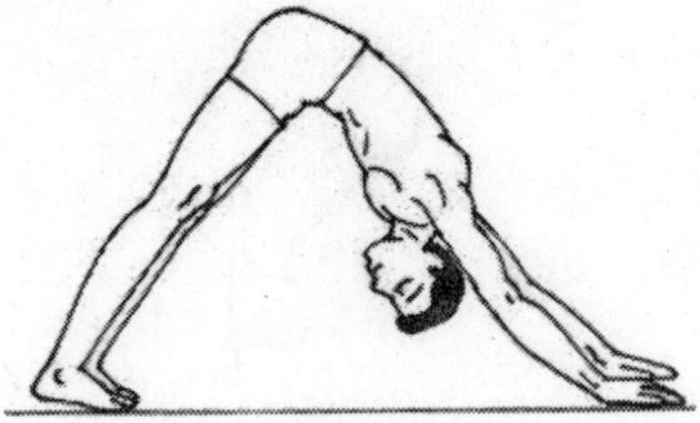

Position IX: Ashwa Sanchalanasana

Procedure: Same as position-IV.

Benefits: Same as position-IV

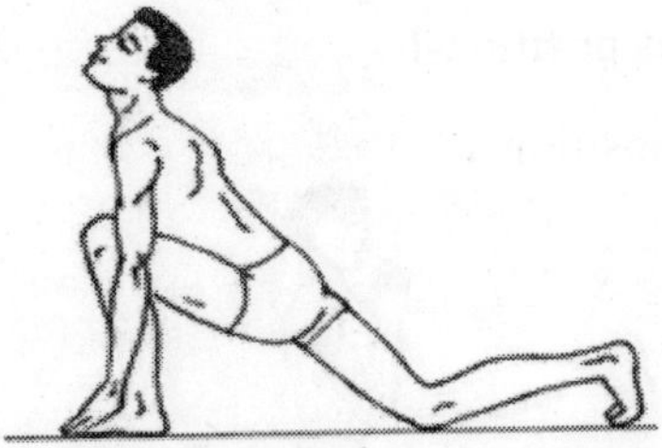

Position X: Padahastasana

Procedure: Same as position-III.

Benefits: Same as position-III.

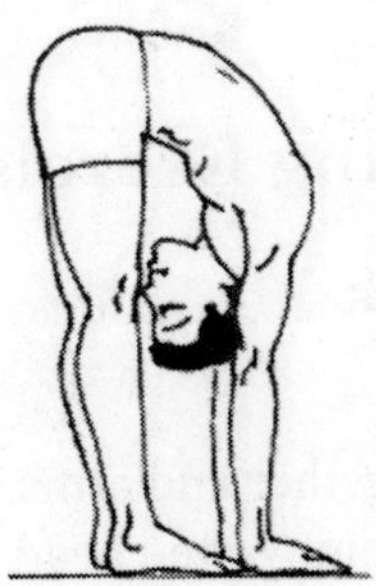

Position XI: Hasta Utthanasana

Procedure: Same as position-II.

Benefits: Same as position-II.

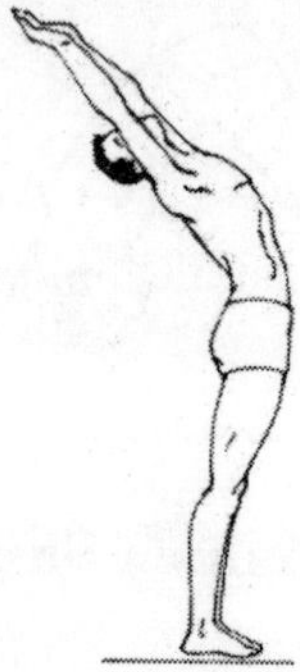

Position XII: Pranamasana

Procedure: Same as position-I.

Benefits: Same as position-I.

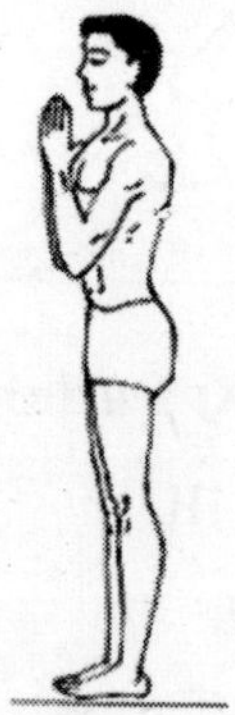

Joint Loosening Exercises Neck-Toes

Griva-Shakti-Vikasak

Procedure

1. Stand with feet together and arms by the side.
2. Exhale and slowly move the head to the right without raising the shoulder.

3. Inhale and return back to initial position.
4. Repeat the same on the left side.

Benefits: Releases tension, heaviness and stiffness in the head, neck and shoulder region.

Kati-Shakti-Vikasak

Procedure

1. Stand with the feet about shoulder width apart and arms by the sides.
2. Raise both the arms forward up to shoulder level with palms facing each other and keep them parallel.
3. While exhaling, twist the body towards the left side so that the right palm touches the left shoulder, and come back with inhalation.
4. Repeat the process on the right side.

Benefits: Releases tension, heaviness and stiffness in the, neck shoulder, arms waist, back and hips.

Jangha-Shakti-Vikasak

Procedure

1. Stand with the feet together arms by the side and palms facing inward.
2. Lift both the arms up to shoulder level, plain facing downwards.
3. Bend the knees and bring down your body to the squatting position.
4. In the final position both the arms and thighs should be parallel to the ground.

Benefits: Releases tension, heaviness and stiffness from the ankle, knee and hip joints.

Padamul-Shakti-Vikasak

Procedure

1. Stand with the feet together and arms by the side.
2. Move your toes upward and hold.

Benefits: Releases tension, heaviness and stiffness in the ankle, knee and strengthen calf and back muscles.

Asanas (Yoga postures)

1. Standing

Ardha Karticakrasana (Half Waist Wheel Pose)

Procedure

1. Stand with the feet about shoulder width apart and arms by the sides.
2. Raise both the arms forward up to shoulder level with palms facing each other and keep the parallel.
3. While exhaling twist the body towards the left sides so that the right palm touches the left shoulder, come back with inhalation.
4. Repeat the process in right side.

Benefits: Releases tension, heaviness and stiffness in the, neck shoulder, arms waist, back and hips.

Ardhachakrasana (Half wheel pose)

Procedure

1. Stand straight with hands on both side and palms should be touching the thighs.
2. Hold the waist by both the hands.
3. Gently bend backwards keeping the arms in line what the ears.
4. Keep the elbows and knees straight.
5. Bend the head and upper trunk slightly backward.

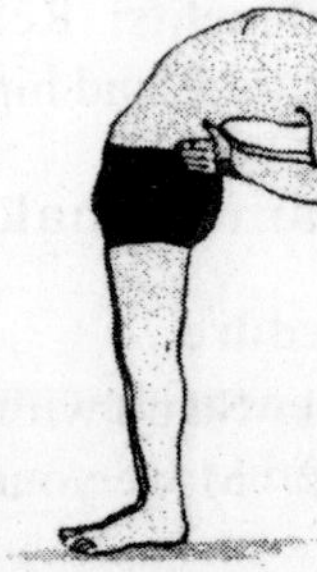

Benefits: Stretches the front upper torso and tones the arms and shoulder muscles. Strengthens neck muscles and lung oxygenations.

Padahastasana (Standing forward bend)

Procedure

1. Bend forward from the hips until the fingers or palms of the hands touch the floor on either side of the feet.
2. Keep the knees straight and bring the forehead as close as possible to the knee.

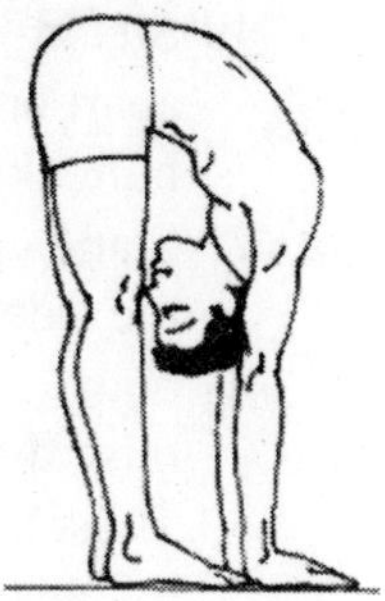

Benefits: Improves digestion, removes flatulence and indigestion. Increase flexibility of the back.

2. Sitting

Paschimottanasana (Seated forward bend pose)

Procedure

1. Sit on the floor with the legs outstretched, feet together and hands on the knees.
2. Slowly bend forward from the hips, sliding the hands down the legs. Try to grasp the big toes with the fingers and thumbs.
3. Move slowly without forcing or jerking. Hold the position for a few seconds. Relax the back and leg muscles, allowing them to gently stretch.
4. Keeping the legs straight and utilizing the arm muscles, not the back muscles, begin to bend the elbows and gently bring the trunk down towards the legs, maintaining a firm grip on the toes, feet or legs.
5. Try to touch the knees with the forehead.

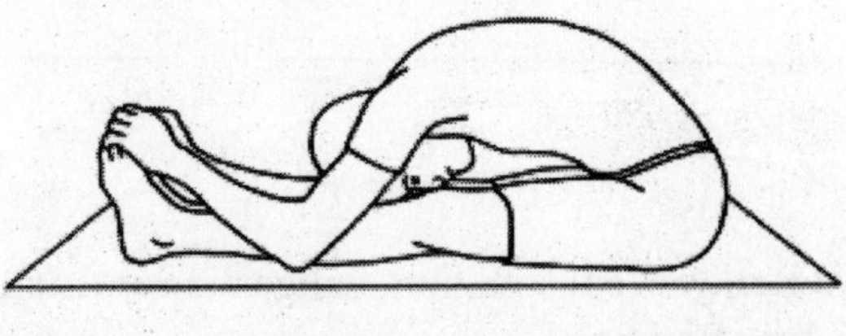

Benefits: Increases flexibility of hip joints. Tones and massages the internal organs. Helps to maintain weight.

Ardha Ustrasana (Half camel pose)

Procedure

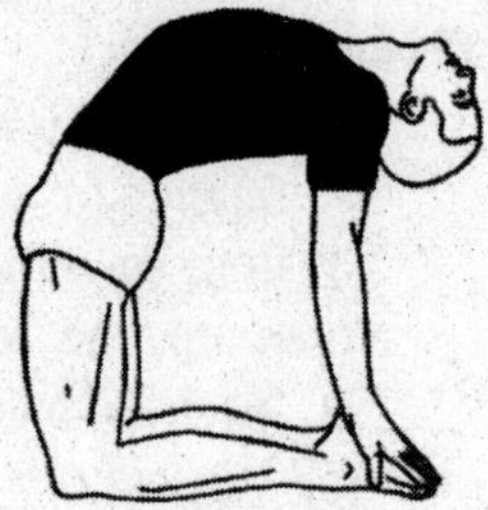

1. Sit in Vajrasana. Move the knees apart and the ankles to the side of the buttocks.
2. Stand up on the knees with the arms at the sides. Keep the feet flat behind the body. Stretch the arms sideways and raise them to shoulder level.
3. Twist to the right, reach back with the right hand and hold the left ankle.
4. Stretch the left arm in front of the head so that the hand is at eyebrow level. The head should be slightly back with the eyes gazing at the raised hand. Push the hips forward in the final position and keep the thighs vertical. Hold this position while comfortable, retaining the gaze on the left hand.

Benefits: Beneficial for the digestive and reproductive systems. Relieving backache, rounded back and drooping shoulders.

Bhujangasana (Cobra pose)

Procedure

1. Lie down on abdomen with legs close together to the ground.
2. Place hands besides the body with palm touching on ground.
3. Lift the prone body from the ground up to the naval region.

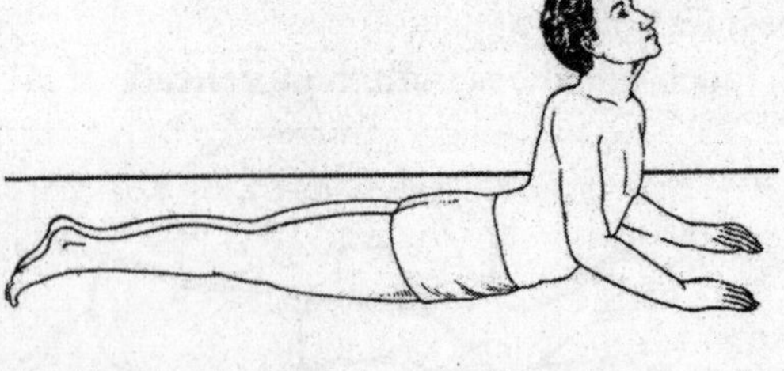

Benefits: Relieves constipation, indigestion and flatulence. Helps in improving lung function.

Salabhasana (Locust pose)

Procedure

1. Lie flat on the stomach with the legs and feet together and the soles of the feet uppermost.
2. The arms placed either under the body or by the sides, with the palms downward or the hands clenched.
3. Stretch the chin slightly forward and rest it on the floor throughout the practice.
4. Close the eyes and relax the body. Slowly raise the legs as high as possible without straining, keeping them straight and together. The elevation of the legs is produced by applying pressure with the arms against the floor and contracting the lower back muscles.

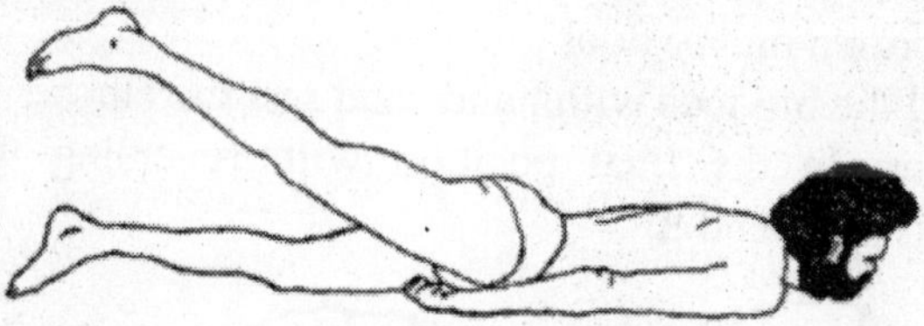

Benefits: Strengthens the lower back and pelvic organs and provides relief from backache, mild sciatica and slipped disc when the condition is not serious. It tones and balances the functioning of the liver, stomach, bowels and other abdominal organs and increases appetite.

Dhanurasana (Bow pose)

Procedure

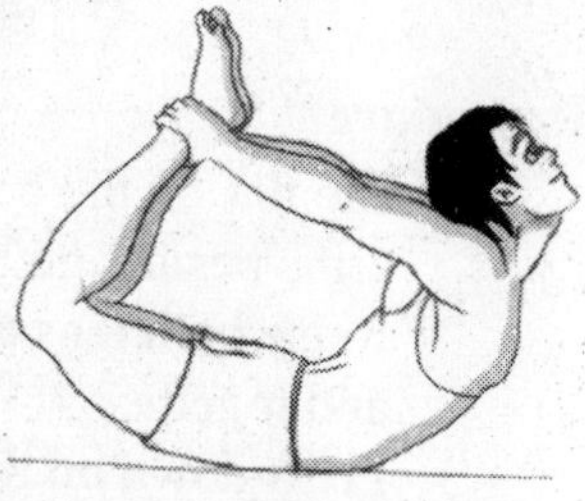

1. Lie flat on the stomach with the legs and feet together and the arms and hands beside the body.
2. Bend the knees and bring the heels close to the buttocks. Clasp the hands around the ankles. Place the chin on the floor.
3. Tense the leg muscles and push the feet away from the body. Arch the back, lifting the thighs, chest and head together.

4. Keep the arms straight. In the final position the head is tilted back and the abdomen supports the entire body on the floor.

Benefits: Messages internal organs thus control their secretion. Increases digestion. Aligns the spinal column increases the strength of the ligaments, muscles and nerves thus removes stiffness. Helps to correct hunching of the upper back. Strengthens leg muscles and improves lung capacities.

Supine pose Matsyasana (Fish pose)

Procedure

1. Sit in Padmasana. Bend backward carefully supporting the body with the arms and elbows. With exhaling, arch the back by lifting the neck and the chest, take the head back and rest the crown on the floor.
2. Hold the big toes with hands and rest the elbows on the floor.
3. Return to the final position with reversing the order of backward bending.

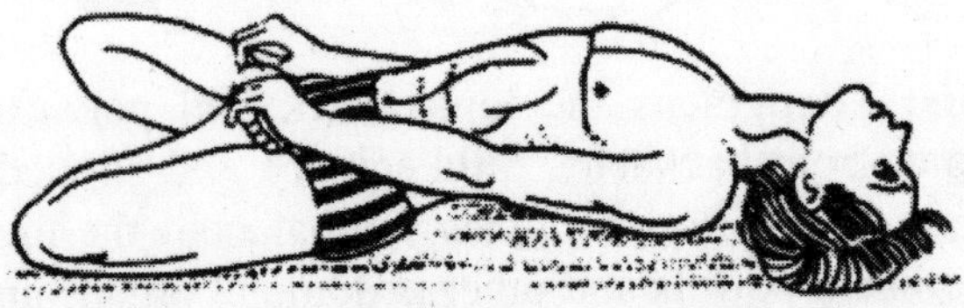

Benefits: Improves digestion and lung capacity. Increases flexibility of shoulder and back. Makes the thyroid, parathyroid and adrenal gland healthy.

Halasana (Plough pose)

Procedure

1. Lie flat on the back with the legs and feet together. Place the arms beside the body with the palms facing down.
2. Raise both legs to the vertical position, keeping them straight and together.
3. Press down on the arms and lift the buttocks, rolling the back away from the floor. Lower the legs over the head. Bring the toes towards the floor behind the head.

4. Turn the palms up, bend the elbows and place the hands behind the ribcage to support the back.
5. Release the hands. Raise the legs up to *Sarvangasanaand* gradually slide down to the floor. Lie flat on the back and relax.

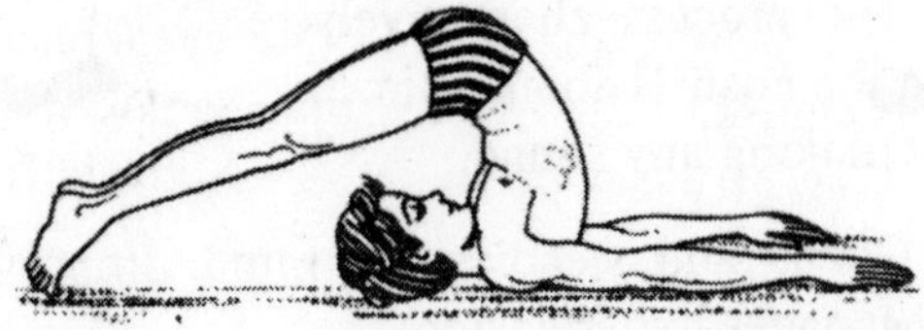

Benefits: Strengthens the back muscle and makes spine flexible. Activates thyroid glands and controls metabolism. Improves digestion and activates pancreas.

Pranayama (Yoga Breathing Techniques) Kapalbhati

Procedure

1. Sit in Padmasana, put both hands on respective knees. Exhale faster and forcibly through both the nostrils. Simultaneously draw the abdomen in.
2. After completing exhalation with force, take the breath in and bring the abdomen in previous position.
3. The sound produced during inhalation and exhalation should be like a bellows of the blacksmith.

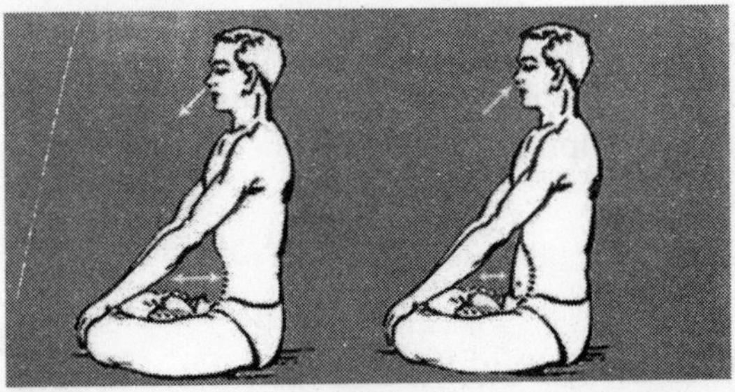

Benefits: Cleanses the naso-pharynx. Improves digestion.

Anulom-Viloma (Alternate Nostril Breathing)

Procedure

1. Sit in Padmasana with head and spine erect and eyes closed.
2. Close the right nostrils with the right thumb.

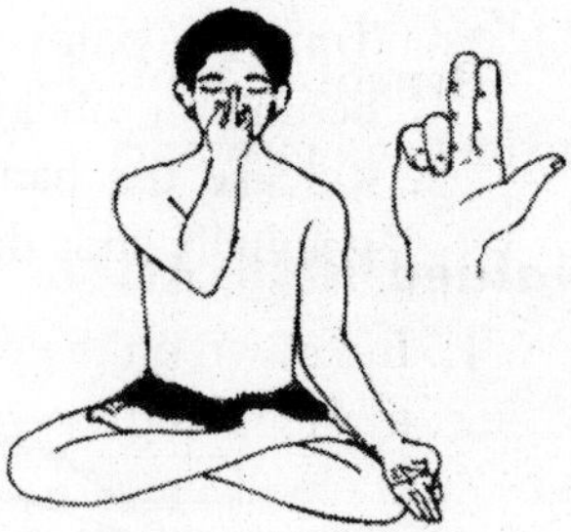

3. Inhale through the left nostril just before closing it with ring finger and release the air through the right nostril.
4. Repeat the process alternatively for both the nostrils about 5 times without making any sound.

Benefits: Calms and steadies the mind. Improves focus and concentration. Manages hypertension.

Bhastrika (bellows type breathing)

Procedure

1. Sit in a comfortable meditation posture with the hands resting on the knees.
2. Keep the head and spine straight, close the eyes and relax the whole body.
3. Take a deep breath in and breathe out forcefully through the nose.
4. Immediately afterwards, breath in with the same force. The force of inhalation and exhalation must be equal.
5. Continue in this manner, counting 10 breaths.
6. Take a deep breath in and breathe out slowly.

Benefits: This practice burns up toxins and helps balance the doshas or humours: kapha, pitta or bile and vata or wind. Increases metabolic rate and improves digestion.

Bhramari

Procedure

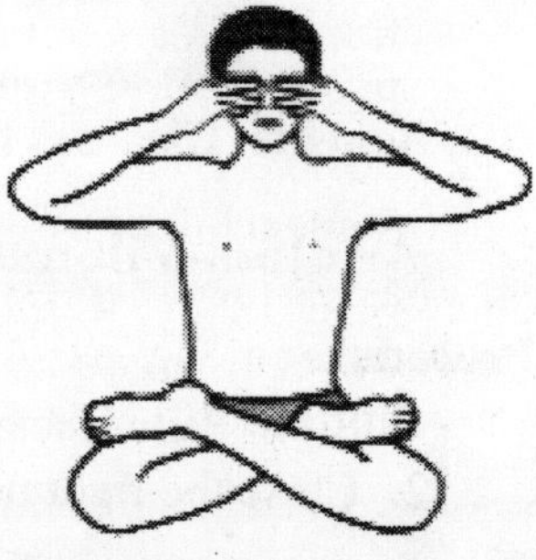

1. Sit in the position of Padmasana.
2. Using both the hands, place index finger on the forehead, close eyes with middle finger and close years with thumbs with lips closed.
3. Inhale deeply and exhale by making a humming sound similar to black bee.

Benefits: Calms the mind and nervous system. Alleviates anger, anxiety and insomnia.

Guided Relaxation

1. Lie down on the ground. Keep a distance of one foot between the legs and keep both the hands open pointing upwards at some distance from the thighs.
2. Close the eyes, keep the neck straight and relax the whole body.
3. Gently inhale and exhale four to five deep breaths.
4. Now observe each part of the body through the mind with resolution and feeling that each part of the body is in a relaxed and stress-free state.
5. Do not sleep during the practice.

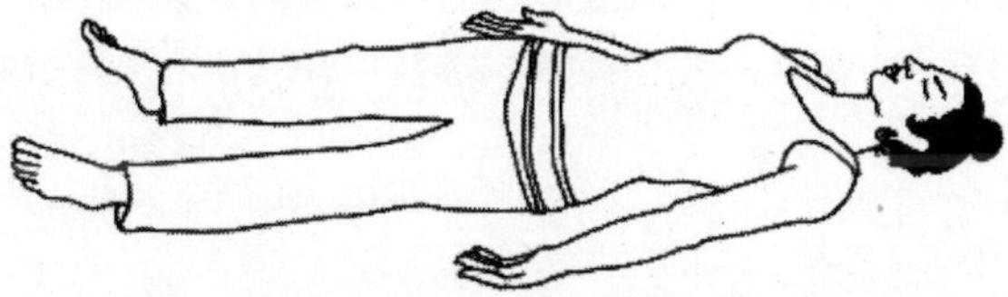

Benefits: Reduces mental stress, depression, high blood pressure, heart diseases and insomnia. The body, mind, brain and soul get complete rest, power, motivation and happiness. The concentration power is developed.

Acknowledgement: Authors are thankful to the Yoga group of DIPAS and Morarji Desai National Institute of Yoga for helpful discussions on different aspects of yogic asanas.

References

1. Tansey WA, Wilson JM, Schaefer KE. Analysis of health data from 10 years of Polaris submarine patrols. Undersea Biomed Res. 1979;6 Suppl:S217-46.
2. Sosiukin AE, Vasiliuk VB, Ivanchenko AV, Saenko SA, Semenchuk OA, Dokhov MA, Verveda AB. [Prognostic assessment for formation of a group of cardiovascular high risk among personnel participating in atomic submarines utilization]. Med Tr Prom Ekol. 2014;(11):6-11.

3. Beare, A. N., K. R. Bondi, R. J. Biersner, and P. Naitoh. 1981. Work and rest on nuclear submarines. Ergonomics. 24: 593-610.
4. Malhotra MS, Wright HC. Arterial air embolism during decompression and its prevention. Proceedings of the Royal Society of London B: Biological Sciences. 1961 Jul 25; 154(956):418-27.

❐

Section III

Yoga as a Non-pharmacological Intervention in Diseases

10
Asthma Management by Yoga

What is Asthma?

Asthma may be described as a chronic lung disease that causes inflammation of the airways and leading to narrowing of the airways. Asthma causes wheezing, chest tightness, breath shortness and coughing. It affects people of all age group, but most often starts during childhood.

Worldwide, more than 300 million people are known to have asthma with 1/10th of those living in India. The prevalence of childhood asthma has continued to increase in last 10 years on the Indian subcontinent.

Symptoms: The symptoms of Asthma may be the following

- It can be mild to moderate to severe.
- Vary from person to person.
- It may flare up from time to time and then not appear for long periods.
- It may vary from one episode to the next.

The cause of Asthma

The actual cause of asthma is not known. However, several reports have shown that there are many factors which can lead to the development of asthma. These factors may include the person's genetics, development of lungs, immune system, and environmental factors/pollution.

How Genetics may cause Asthma?

There is no clear identification of the genes that are involved in causing asthma so far, however it is believed that asthma may be inherited from parents to the offsprings. Atopic diseases such as atopic dermatitis, allergic rhinitis, hay fever and asthma are commonly found within families. Therefore it is speculated that asthma is a disease which can be inherited.

Development of Lungs during Childhood

The early years of a child's life is important when a baby may become susceptible to asthma due to abnormal development of lungs. Premature birth is also one cause where a baby does not have fully developed lungs and is at risk for developing asthma. Premature children are therefore more susceptible to cold and respiratory infections. Exposure to smoke may damage the lungs.

Role of Immune System

The immune system of asthmatic patients develop exaggerated response to certain foreign substances or allergens. The immune cells such as mast cells and basophils recognize these allergen via IgE receptors and get sensitized. When the next episode of allergen exposure occurs to these cells, a hypersensitive response triggers leading to release inflammatory mediators (e.g. histamine) that quickly travel throughout the body causes swelling and narrowing of the airways in the lung. Mediators released by the re-exposure to an allergen also stimulate other kinds of immune cells called eosinophils. Eosinophils contain substances that when released normally fight off parasitic infections, but in asthma, the cells damage the lung causing more inflammation and worsening symptoms. Increased inflammation and obstruction of airflow may be more severe than what is seen during the early phase.

Asthma may be triggered by certain allergens such as

- Dust mites, specifically mite feces, which are coated with enzymes that contain a powerful allergen. These are the primary allergens in the home.
- Animal dander.
- Molds/fungal spores.

- Asthma can be triggered by cockroach feces, saliva and body parts.
- Pollen grains.
- Food additives such as colors may also trigger asthma.

Environmental Factors/Pollutants

Environmental factors/pollution play important role in aggravating asthma. An asthma attack can also be induced or aggravated by direct irritants to the lungs. Important irritants involved in asthma include cigarette smoke, indoor chemicals, and air pollution. The increased air pollution level such as ozone level is directly related to asthma attacks. It causes irritation to the lung air ways. Ozone can reduce lung function and make it more difficult for deep breathing.

Scientific Evidences on Yoga for benefitting in Asthma

A study published by Karam et al. (2017) reported that a simple program of breathing exercises was effective and could be completed in less than 10 minutes per day. For this study they have enrolled 74 patients. The intervention improved breathing for 52.9% of the subjects, while 67.6% felt that their daily activity was improved and 66.1% noted that the exercises allowed decreased use of a rescue inhaler. Most subjects (80.9%) recommended breathing exercises as a complementary therapy for asthma. Overall, Asthma Control Test (ACT) scores improved significantly with a statistically non-significant improvement in Asthma Quality of Life Questionnaire (AQLQ) scores. Rao et. al (2014) reported the efficacy of naturopathy and yoga in bronchial asthma. In this study authors have analyzed 159 bronchial asthma patients, undergoing the naturopathy and yoga programme. Their study found the beneficial effect of combining naturopathy and yoga for the management of bronchial asthma. Khanam et al (1996) studied nine diagnosed bronchial asthma patients. Yoga training was given for seven days in a camp in Adhyatma Sadhna Kendra, New Delhi. The results indicated the reduction in sympathetic reactivity and improvement in the pulmonary ventilation by way of relaxation of voluntary inspiratory and expiratory muscles. The comprehensive yogic life style change programme for patients of Bronchial Asthma has shown significant benefit even within a short period. Agnihotri et al. (2014) evaluated the effect of yoga on biochemical profile of asthmatic patients. The study concluded that the yoga group got significantly better improvement in biochemical variables than the control group. Results showed that yoga can be practiced as adjuvant therapy with standard inhalation therapy for better outcome of asthma. Bidwell et al. (2012) reported that Yoga training improves quality of life in women with asthma. Nagarathna and Nagendra (1985) studied 53 patients with asthma who underwent training for two weeks in an integrated set of yoga exercises, including breathing exercises, suryanamaskar, yogasana (physical postures), pranayama (breath slowing techniques), dhyana (meditation), and a devotional session, and were told to practise these exercises for 65 minutes daily. They were then compared with a control group of 53 patients with asthma matched for age, sex, and type and severity of asthma, who continued to take their usual drugs. There was a significantly greater improvement in the group who practised yoga in the weekly number of attacks of asthma, scores for drug treatment, and peak flow rate. This study showed the efficacy of yoga in the long term management of bronchial asthma. Singh et al. (1990) studied the effects of two pranayama yoga breathing exercises on airway reactivity, airway calibre, symptom scores, and medication use in patients with mild asthma in a randomised, double-blind, placebo-controlled, crossover trial. After baseline assessment over 1 week, 18 patients with mild asthma practised slow deep breathing for 15 min twice a day for two consecutive 2-week periods. During the active period, subjects were asked to breathe through a Pink City Lung (PCL) exerciser-a device which imposes slowing of breathing and a 1:2 inspiration: expiration duration ratio equivalent to pranayama breathing methods; during the control period, subjects breathed through a matched placebo device. Mean forced expiratory volume in 1 s (FEV1), peak expiratory flow rate, symptom score, and inhaler use over the last 3 days of each treatment period were assessed in comparison with the baseline assessment period; all improved more with the PCL exerciser than with the placebo device, but the differences were not significant. There was a significant increase in the dose of histamine needed to provoke a 20% reduction in FEV1 (PD20) during pranayama breathing but not with the placebo device. Jain et al. (1991) studied forty six young asthmatics with a history of childhood asthma who were admitted for yoga training. Parameters measured were resting pulmonary functions, exercise capacity, and exercise-induced bronchial lability index. Yoga training resulted in a significant increase in pulmonary function and exercise capacity. A follow-up study spanning two years showed a good response with reduced symptom score and drug requirements in these subjects. The study concluded that yoga training is beneficial for young asthmatics.

A number of yoga intervention studies have been reported on asthmatic patients.

Asanas for Management of Asthma: Some Asanas and Pranayam which are helpful in Asthma management are given below:

Ardha Chakrasan

Procedure

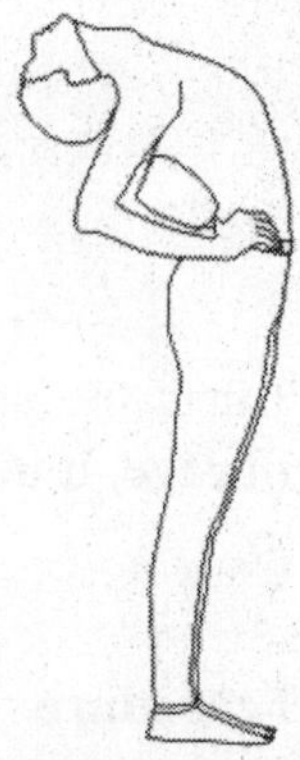

1. Stand straight with feet together and arms alongside the body.
2. Balance your weight equally on both feet.
3. Breathing in, extend your arms overhead, palms facing each other.
4. Breathing out, gently bend backwards pushing the pelvis forward, keeping the arms in line with the ears, elbows and knees straight, head up, and lifting your chest towards the ceiling.
5. Hold. Breathing in, come back up.
6. Breathing out, bring the arms down and relax.

Benefits: Bending backswords gives room to breathe and thus helps respiratory system and can relieve Asthma problems.

Supta Vajrasan

Procedure

1. Sit in Vajrasana. Placing the palms on the floor beside the buttocks, fingers pointing to the front.
2. Slowly bend backward, placing the right forearm and the elbow on the ground and then the left.
3. Bring the crown of the head to the ground while arching the back. Place the hands on the thighs.
4. Try to keep the lower legs in contact with the floor. If necessary, separate the knees.

5. Make sure that you are not overstraining the muscles and ligaments of the legs.
6. Close the eyes and relax the body. Breathe deeply and slowly in the final position.
7. Release in the reverse order, breathing in and taking the support of the elbows and the arms raise the head above the ground.
8. Then shift the body weight on the left arm and elbow by sliding the body, then slowly coming to the starting position.
9. Never leave the final position by straightening the legs first; it may dislocate the knee joints.

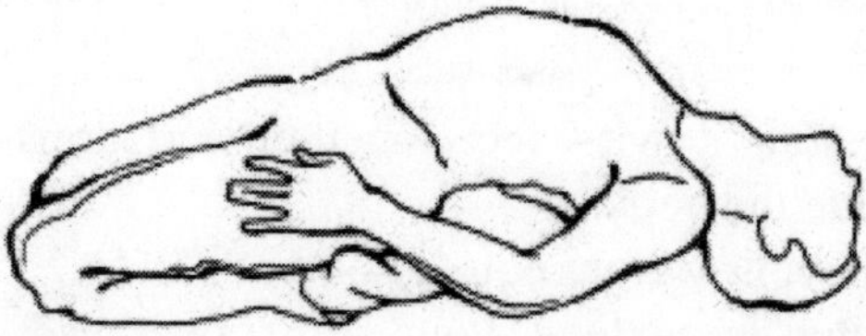

Benefits: Benefits in asthma, bronchitis and other lung ailments. Tones the spinal nerves, neck and back muscles and stretches the ribcage. It increases lung capacity.

Bhujangasan

Procedure

1. Lie down on abdomen with legs close together to the ground.
2. Place hands besides the body with palm touching on ground. Lift the prone body from the ground up to the naval region.

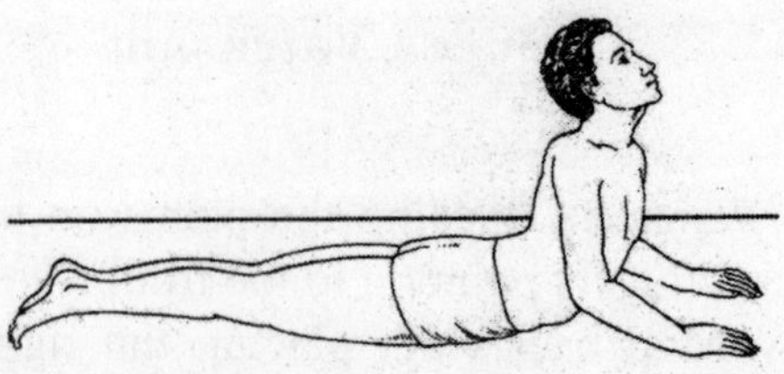

Benefits: Beneficial in asthmaas the lungs and chest cavity is expanded during Bhujangasan. Regular practice over a period of time may eliminate the use of medication for asthma patients.

Halasana

Procedure

1. Lie flat on your back, with your arms placed beside your body and your palms facing downwards.
2. Inhale, and lift your feet off the ground using your abdominal muscles. Your legs should be at a 90-degree angle.
3. Use your hands to support your hips and lift them off the floor.
4. Bring your feet in at a 180-degree angle, such that your toes are placed over and beyond your head.
5. Make sure your back is perpendicular to the ground.
6. Hold the position for a minute while focusing on your breathing. Exhale, and gently bring down your legs. Avoid jerking your legs while releasing the pose.

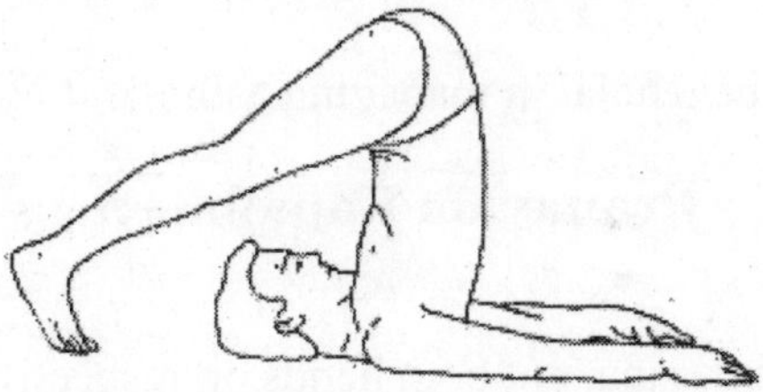

Benefits: Stretches the shoulders and improves flexibility of spine, flushes mucous, strengthens the lungs and increases the immunity and beneficial in asthma. This pose balances the spleen and the liver and increases the digestion and absorption activities properly, balances the secretion of pancreas and protects the body and kidney gets strengthened and refreshed. Since it strengthens the liver the Red Blood Corpuscles are increased and make you feel active.

Sirsasana

Procedure

1. Sit on the mat and kneel down.
2. Join the fingers and keep your hands on the mat as like a triangle.
3. Keep down your top of the head on the mat and hold it.
4. Press your head, elbow, finger on the mat and lift your knees upward. At the same time bring your legs front and make the spinal cord straightly.

5. This is the Artha Sirsasana pose. Practice this asana for one month at the beginning stage. Minimum fifty to hundred counts enough at the starting period.
6. Lift your legs upward, and put your heels on the wall make the spine straight then count hundred.
7. After practicing this for three months then do the asana without the support of wall.
8. Bring your legs down by folding the knees, press your foot and elbow then bring your head up and sit on your knees.
9. Then lie down on the mat in Savasana and relax.

Benefits: Sirsasana also ensures healthier and more effective lung tissue. When standing or sitting upright, gravity pulls our fluids earthward and blood perfuses the lower lungs more thoroughly. When we invert, blood perfuses the well-ventilated upper lobes of the lungs, thus ensuring more efficient oxygen-to-blood exchange and healthier lung tissue.

This pose is beneficial in managing asthma.

Pranayam Kapalbhati

Procedure

1. Sit in Padmasana, put both hands on respective knees. Exhale faster and forcibly through both the nostrils. Simultaneously draw the abdomen in.
2. After completing exhalation with force, take the breath in and bring the abdomen in previous position.
3. The sound produced during inhalation and exhalation should be like a bellows of the blacksmith.

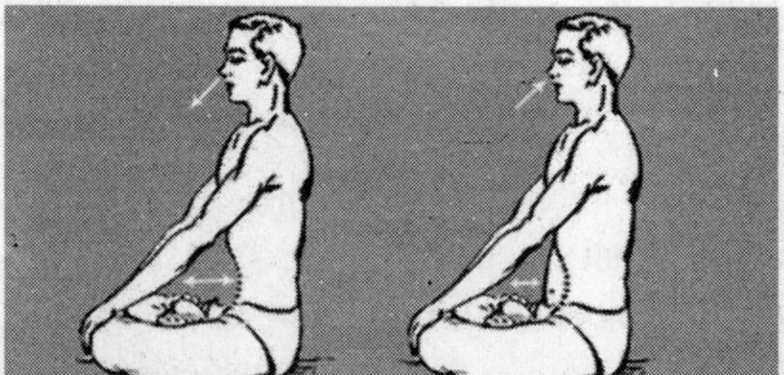

Benefits: The lungs capacity to hold the oxygen increases. Practising Kapalabhati leads to good circulation of oxygen throughout the body and as a results helps in asthma, and common cold.

Bhastrika (bellows type beathing)

Procedure

1. Sit in a comfortable meditation posture with the hands resting on the knees.
2. Keep the head and spine straight, close the eyes and relax the whole body.
3. Take a deep breath in and breathe out forcefully through the nose.
4. Immediately afterwards, breath in with the same force. The force of inhalation and exhalation must be equal.
5. Continue in this manner, counting 10 breaths.
6. Take a deep breath in and breathe out slowly.

Benefits: In Bhastrika, breath is exhaled forcibly and quickly. One should inhale and exhale breath like a blower. In this Pranayam, blood flow occurs upward during rapid inhalation and downward during rapid exhalation. This is the only Pranayam which removes all ailments related to vata, pitta and kapha. It is very good for one's mental and physical health. It cures depression, tiredness, insomnia, phobia and anxiety. It is beneficial in asthma.

Suryabhedhaka Pranayam

Procedure

1. Sit comfortably in cross-legged position, with eyes closed.
2. Make the Pranayam mudra with your right hand and close your left nostril with your little finger and ring finger.
3. Exhale slowly from your right nostril (called the 'surya nadi' in yogic terminology); then inhale as deeply as you can, with sound, with the same nostril.
4. Now do Jalandhar bandh and Mulbandh, (Jalandhar Bandh – pressurize muscles of neck and bend chin forward, Mulbandh-rectum is held upward) and press your stomach inside. Stay in this position as long as possible, then release bandh and exhale very slowly through the left nostril (called 'chander nari').
5. This is one round of Suryabhedi Pranayam. Repeat 8 to 10 times. Beginners should do this Pranayam without holding the breath.

Benefits: It is helpful in cold cough and asthma. It give energy to the body. This Pranayam is very helpful in cold climate.

Ujjayi Pranayam

Procedure

1. Sit comfortably in cross-legged position, with eyes closed, inhale deeply, and then exhale. Tighten your neck muscles and make a sound with your closed mouth, while inhaling.
2. When lungs are full, practice Jalandhar bandh, Mulbandh and Uddiayan bandh while holding your breath for as long as you can. (Mulbandh — rectum is held upward. Uddiyan Bandh — hold stomach inward and Jalandhar Bandh — pressurize muscles of neck and bend chin forward). Then release bandh and make Pranayam mudra with your right hand and close your right nostril. Now exhale with your left nostril very slowly.
3. This is one round of Ujjayi Pranayam. It can be repeated for 10 times. Beginners should do this Pranayam without holding the breath.

Benefits: Ujjayi pranayama not only heats the body but it also helps to sooth and calm the mind, clears the throat, removes cough, cures snoring. It is beneficial in Asthma.

Note: It is very useful in heart disease, but heart patient needs to practice it without holding the breath.

References

1. Karam M, Kaur BP, Baptist AP. A modified breathing exercise program for asthma is easy to perform and effective. J Asthma. 2017 Mar; 54 (2): 217-222.
2. Rao YC, Kadam A, Jagannathan A, Babina N, Rao R, Nagendra HR. Efficacy of naturopathy and yoga in bronchial asthma. Indian J Physiol Pharmacol. 2014 Jul-Sep; 58 (3): 233-9.
3. Khanam AA, Sachdeva U, Guleria R, Deepak KK. Study of pulmonary and autonomic functions of asthma patients after yoga training. Indian J Physiol Pharmacol.1996 Oct; 40(4):318-24.

4. Agnihotri S, Kant S, Kumar S, Mishra RK, Mishra SK. Impact of yoga on biochemical profile of asthmatics: A randomized controlled study. Int J Yoga. 2014 Jan; 7(1):17-21.
5. Nagarathna R, Nagendra HR. Yoga for bronchial asthma: a controlled study. Br Med J (Clin Res Ed). 1985 Oct 19; 291(6502):1077-9.
6. Singh V, Wisniewski A, Britton J, Tattersfield A. Effect of yoga breathing exercises (pranayama) on airway reactivity in subjects with asthma. Lancet. 1990 Jun 9; 335(8702):1381-3.
7. Jain SC, Rai L, Valecha A, Jha UK, Bhatnagar SO, Ram K. Effect of yoga training on exercise tolerance in adolescents with childhood asthma. J Asthma.1991; 28(6):437-42.

❐

11
Yoga Fights Obesity and Eating Disorders

India has the second highest number of obese children in the world after China. Around 14.4 million kids in the country have excess weight. Globally, over two billion children and adults suffer from health problems related to being overweight or obese, and an increasing percentage of people die from these health conditions.

What is Obesity?

Overweight and obesity are defined as abnormal or excessive fat accumulation that presents a risk to health. A crude population measure of obesity is the body mass index (BMI), a person's weight (in kilograms) divided by the square of his or her height (in metres). An ideal body mass index (BMI) is 18.5-24.9 kg/m^2 for both sexes. A BMI between 25 and 29.9 kg/m^2 is considered overweight and that of 30 kg/m^2 and above defines obesity. This applies to adults, aged 18 years and above. The prevalence of obesity in India is 2-15 per cent in urban, and 0-6 per cent in rural population by using current definition of obesity (BMI > 30 kg/m^2).

In India women suffer from a dual burden of malnutrition with nearly half of them being either too thin or overweight. National Family Health Survey-3 (NFHS-3) study undertaken at the national level during the year 2006, revealed that the percentage of ever married women in the age group of 15-49 years who are overweight or obese increased from 11 percent in NFHS-2 to 15 in the NFHS-3. Overweight and obesity were found to be more than 3 times higher in urban than in rural areas.

Overweight and obesity are major risk factors for a number of chronic diseases, including diabetes, cardiovascular diseases and cancer. Obesity has reached epidemic proportions globally, with at least 2.8 million people dying every year as a result of being overweight or obese. Once associated with high-income countries, obesity is now also prevalent in low- and middle-income countries.

BMI Classification	
Underweight	< 18.5
Normal range	18.5-24.9
Overweight	≥ 25.0
Obese	≥ 30

Prevention of Obesity

The children generally become overweight or obese because they don't get enough physical activity in combination with poor eating habits. The lifestyle and genetics also contribute to a child's weight status.

Falling under both the categories (obesity and overweight) can cause serious disorders in the human body. To prevent obesity, one should keep in mind to remove the things that are harmful to the health and adding the things that are beneficial for the health. To start with, you should first have an ideal diet and also do yoga/physical exercise.

What are the steps which help prevent overweight and obesity during childhood and adolescence? They include:

1. Change family eating habits and activity levels gradually rather than focusing on weight.
2. Change the habits and the weight will take care of itself.
3. Try to be a role model. Parents who eat healthy foods and regularly do yoga and exercise may set an example that increases the likelihood their children will do the same.
4. Encourage Yoga and exercise. Children should have an hour of yoga and exercise most days of the week. More than an hour of activity may promote weight loss and subsequent maintenance.
5. Reduce time in front of the TV and computer to less than two hours a day.

6. Encourage children to eat only when hungry, and to eat slowly.
7. Avoid using food as a reward or withholding food as a punishment.
8. Keep the refrigerator stocked with fat-free or low-fat milk and fresh fruit and vegetables instead of soft drinks and snacks high in sugar and fat.
9. Serve at least five servings of fruits and vegetables daily.
10. Encourage children to drink water rather than beverages with added sugar, such as soft drinks, sports drinks and fruit juice drinks.

Prevention of Obesity by Yoga

Yoga is a technique that always has an aim to promote the holistic living. There are some asanas and pranayama that a person can do in order to reduce obesity.

1. **Paschimottanasan:** It helps to massage the organs located at the abdominal and the pelvic region and help in improving digestion effectively in order to reduce obesity.

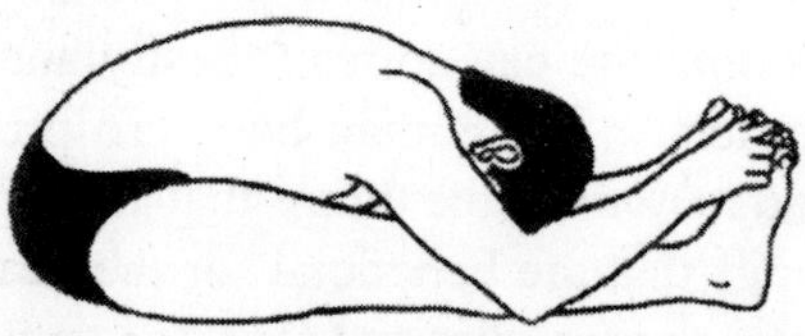

2. **Veerbhadrasan:** It helps to improve the balancing skill of a person and also builds up their stamina. Practicing this asana leads to stimulation of the abdominal organs.

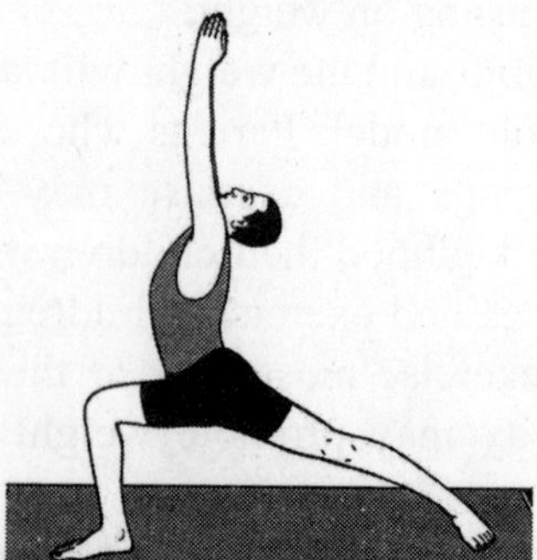

3. **Dandasana:** Practicing this pose helps to tone the abdomen region and is beneficial for the upper body parts by strengthening the wrists as well as arms.

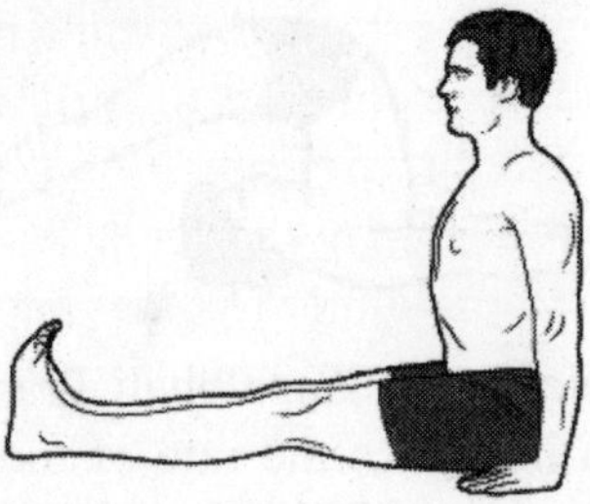

4. **Poorvottanasana:** Practicing this pose is very good for the intestine and the organs located at abdominal region as it stretches the intestine and organs at abdominal region and also tones the abdomen.

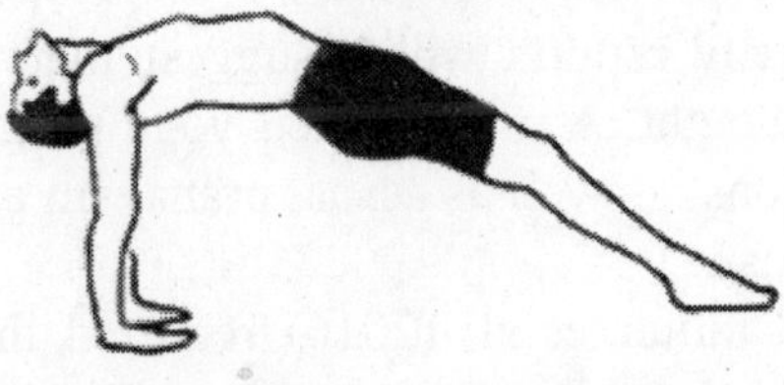

5. **Naukasana:** Practicing this pose helps in strengthening muscles of the abdominal region, improving digestion and stimulating the intestine.

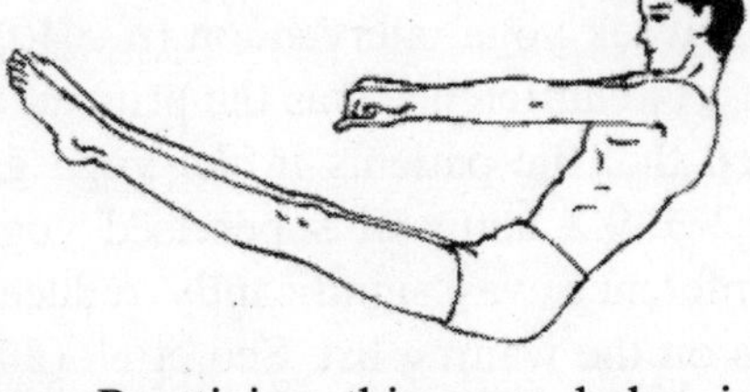

6. **Shalabhasana:** Practicing this pose helps in massaging and toning the organs at the abdominal region and also improves digestion and flexibility.

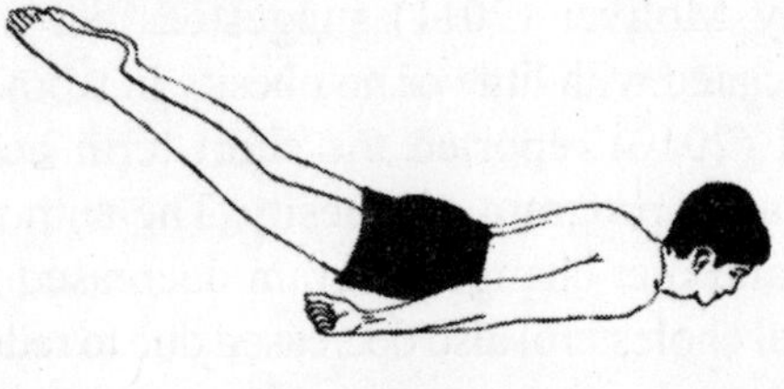

7. **Halasana:** Practicing this pose helps in strengthening the muscles located at the abdominal region and prevents stress and fatigue.

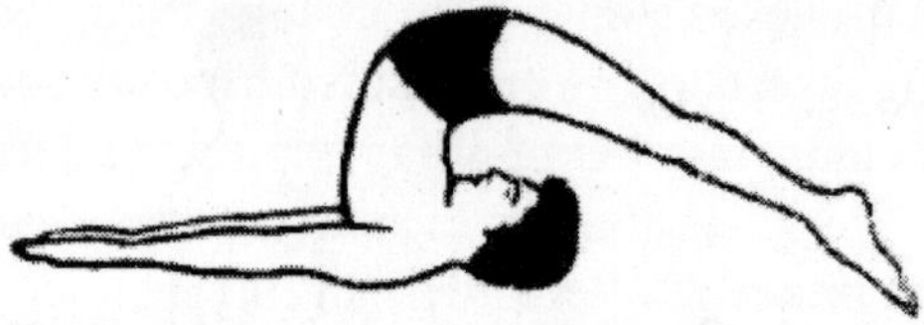

8. **Kapalbhati Pranayama:** Kapalbhati Pranayama is a breathing technique, which increases the rate of metabolism and helps in reducing accumulation of fat. Therefore it results in reducing the overweight. This pranayama also improves GI Tract functioning, absorption and assimilation of food components.

Scientific Evidences of Yoga in Prevention of Obesity

There are many reports which suggest that yoga can prevent obesity and overweight. A multifaceted yoga program that includes dietary modifications, as well as asana, pranayam and meditation can facilitate weight loss.

In a study, Cramer et al. (2016) reported that 12-week yoga intervention had moderately strong positive effects on anthropometric and self-reported variables in women with abdominal obesity. In this study, 60 women with abdominal obesity (waist circumference ≥ 88 cm; body-mass index [BMI] ≥ 25) were randomly allocated in a 2:1 ratio to either a 12-week yoga intervention (n = 40) or a waiting list (n = 20). The waist circumference was the primary endpoint. Results obtained suggested that the patients in the yoga group participated in a mean of 30.2 ± 9.2 hours of supervised yoga practice. Their abdominal circumference was significantly reduced in comparison to the participants on the waiting list. Seo et al. (2012) reported that an 8-week of yoga training improves body composition in obese adolescent boys, suggesting that yoga training may be effective in controlling some metabolic syndrome factors in obese adolescent boys. A study by Moliver (2011) suggested that a long-term yoga practice was associated with little or no obesity in women over 45 years.

Telles et. al (2010) reported the short term health impact of a yoga and diet change program on obesity. The authors were reported that 6-day yoga and diet change program decreased the BMI and the fat-free mass. Total cholesterol also decreased due to reduced HDL levels.

Eating Disorders and Management by Yoga

Eating disorders: Eating disorders are abnormal attitude towards food that causes someone to change their eating habits and behaviour. Eating disorders are one of the unspoken secrets that affect many families. A large number of urban adolescent and young women are afflicted with this disorder, however, no authentic data available on the prevalence of this type of disorders in Indians.

What is the Cause of Eating Disorder?

The modelling industry, TV, films and magazines, put the images of ideal women as unrealistically thin, which causes some women to lose social and psychological confidence in them. The young women trying to emulate these models and they attempt to regain it by disordered eating behaviours. Researchers believe that the growing number of eating disorders might be attributable to the mass media. Aggressive advertising by the diet and cosmetic industries is generally recognized as contributing factors towards eating disorders.

Types of Eating Disorder

Mainly three of the most common eating disorders are:

1. **Anorexia nervosa:** This disorder occurs most commonly in adolescent females, characterized by abnormal body image, fear of obesity, and prolonged refusal to eat, sometimes resulting in death.
2. **Bulimia:** Serious disorder, especially common in adolescents and young women, marked by excessive eating, often followed by self-induced vomiting, purging or fasting.
3. **Binge Eating Disorder:** It is characterized by an uncontrolled consumption of large quantities of food in a short period of time, even if person does not feel hungry.

Treatment of Eating Disorder

Treatment of eating disorders is available, although recovering from an eating disorder can take long time. It is important for the person affected to want to get better and support of family and friends is invaluable. Three goals characterize the treatment of anorexia nervosa: (1) weight gain, (2) changed attitudes toward food and eating and (3) resolution of underlying personal and family conflicts.

Unfortunately, therapeutic intervention is not always successful and the condition may persist for years. Recovering from bulimia includes stopping binge-purge cycles and regaining control over eating behavior. Psychological counseling may be helpful. People with binge eating disorder should get help from a health professional which could include instruction in how to keep track of and change unhealthy eating behaviors, identify social factors that contribute to the problem, psychological counseling, and medications.

Scientific Evidences of Yoga in Treating Eating Disorder

Yoga interventions increase self-awareness through Asanas, Pranayam and Meditation. The mindfulness techniques of yoga may be helpful in treating eating disorders. There are several reports published in scientific journals that Yoga practices may be used as adjunct therapy for the treatment of eating disorders. In a recently published study Pacanowski et al. (2017) reported that Yoga significantly reduced pre-meal negative effect, an eating disorders risk factor. Klein and Cook-Cottone (2013) published a review on effects of yoga on eating disorder, they found that Yoga practitioners were reported to be at decreased risk for eating disorders, and eating disorder risk and symptoms were reduced or unchanged after yoga interventions. Daubenmier, (2005) examined how practicing yoga affects body awareness, body responsiveness, and body satisfaction. Total 138 women were participated in this study. The study was divided in three groups: a yoga group, an aerobic exercisers group, and a control group. Participants were given surveys that measured body awareness, body satisfaction, and eating disorder symptoms. It was found that the yoga group reported lower scores on all measures associated with eating disorder behaviors, including greater body awareness when compared with non-yoga practitioners. The results indicated that yoga decreases eating disorder risk factors at higher rates than other forms of exercise. Regular practice of yoga may facilitate healthy eating behaviors. Yoga practitioners may regulate food intake based on bodily needs rather emotional or other factors. In line with this reasoning, Kristeller and Hallett (1999) found that participation in a 6-week meditation-based inter-vention reduced the number and severity of binges among obese women diagnosed with binge eating disorder. In addition, in a randomized study, Telch, *et al.*, (2001) found that dialectical behavior therapy, which fosters mindful awareness of moment-to-moment experience, reduced binge eating and eating pathology in participants diagnosed with binge eating disorder compared to a wait-list control condition (Daubenmier, 2005).

Yoga may be helpful in treating eating disorder recovery by access memories, messages, and wisdom stored in the body. The ultimate goal of recovery is in fact yoga re-connecting and integrating all parts of the self to live a more perceptive, peaceful, and soulful life.

References

1. Cramer H, Thoms MS, Anheyer D, Lauche R, Dobos G. Yoga in Women With Abdominal Obesity a Randomized Controlled Trial. Dtsch Arztebl Int. 2016 Sep 30;113(39):645-652.
2. Seo DY, Lee S, Figueroa A, Kim HK, Baek YH, Kwak YS, Kim N, Choi TH, Rhee BD, Ko KS, Park BJ, Park SY, Han J. Yoga training improves metabolic parameters in obese boys. Korean J Physiol Pharmacol. 2012 Jun;16(3):175-80.
3. Moliver N, Mika E, Chartrand M, Burrus S, Haussmann R, Khalsa S. Increased Hatha yoga experience predicts lower body mass index and reduced medication use in women over 45 years. Int J Yoga. 2011 Jul;4(2):77-86.
4. Telles S, Naveen VK, Balkrishna A, Kumar S. Short term health impact of a yoga and diet change program on obesity. Med Sci Monit. 2010 Jan;16(1):CR35-40.
5. Pacanowski CR, Diers L, Crosby RD, Neumark-Sztainer D. Yoga in the treatment of eating disorders within a residential program: A randomized controlled trial. Eat Disord. 2017 Jan-Feb;25(1):37-51.
6. Klein J, Cook-Cottone C. The effects of yoga on eating disorder symptoms and correlates: a review. Int J Yoga Therap. 2013; (23): 41-50.
7. Daubenmier JJ. The relationship of yoga, body awareness, and body responsiveness to self-objectification and disordered eating. Psychology of Women Quarterly. 2005; 29: 207–219. Telch C, Agras W., Linehan, M. Dialectical behavior therapy for binge eating disorder. Journal of Consulting and Clinical Psychology. 2001; 69: 1061–1065.

❐

12
Yoga for Better Sleep

Sleep is defined as the natural periodic state of rest for body and mind with closed eyes and partial or complete loss of consciousness. Depth and pattern of sleep is not at all constant, it varies from person to person with stages of sleep and age. During sleep, most of the physiological functions are reduced to basal level and responsiveness to external stimuli decreases. The sleep requirement is not constant and is highest in newborn infants (18-20 hrs), where in case of growing children, adults and old persons it is 12 to 14 hours, 7 to 9 hours and 5 to 7 hours respectively.

Physiological Changes During Sleep

The human body undergoes various changes during different stages of sleep that includes changes in brain wave activity, plasma volume, breathing, body temperature, heart rate and other physiological functions. The probable reason behind the changes is decreased physiological demands. Some of the major changes are listed below:

Brain Activity: For centuries, researchers believed sleep, as a period of brain inactivity, yet research over the last 65 years has shown that the brain remains active during sleep although progressive decrease in the "firing" rate of most neurons is reported. Electrical activity of brain varies with the stages of sleep.

Plasma Volume: Plasma volume is reported to be decrease by about 10% during sleep.

Cardiovascular Activity: One of the major goals of sleep is to give the heart a chance to rest from the constant demands of waking life. During sleep, the heart rate reduces from 72 to 60-45 beats per minute. Systolic pressure decreases and lowest level is reached about 4th hour of sleep and remains at this level till a short time before waking up. Although during disturbed sleep by exciting dreams, the systolic pressure is elevated to above 130 mm Hg.

Respiratory system: During sleep rate the force of respiration are decreased and respiration becomes irregular.

Body Temperature: During sleep, the central set temperature of our body (98.4°0 F) is reduced by 1 to 2°F. As a result, body uses less energy maintaining its own temperature.

Gastrointestinal tract: Salivary secretion decreases slightly during sleep. Gastric secretion remains unaltered.

Muscle tone: Tone in all the muscles of body decreases very much during sleep. It is called sleep paralysis. Although tone in ocular muscles remain unaltered.

Reflexes: During sleep, certain reflexes particularly knee jerk, are abolished. During deep sleep the Babinski sign becomes positive. A person who has a positive Babinski's reflex will also have in coordination, weakness, and difficulty with muscle control. The Babinski reflex occurs after the sole of the foot has been firmly stroked. The big toe then moves upward or toward the top surface of the foot. Threshold for most of the reflexes increases up to a certain level. Pupils are usually constricted and eyeballs move up and down.

Types and Stages of Sleep

There are two different sleep types:

1. Rapid eye movement sleep (REM sleep)
2. Non-rapid eye movement sleep (NREM sleep or non-REM sleep).

Rapid eye movement sleep (REM sleep): Rapid eye movement sleep is defined as the type of sleep associated with rapid conjugate and frequent movements of the eye balls. Though the eye balls move, it is a kind of deep sleep. This type is also known as paradoxical sleep and occupies almost 30% of total sleeping period. Dreams occur only during this period. REM sleep is considered to be very important because, memory consolidation occurs during this period. During REM sleep electroencephalogram (EEG) shows desynchronized irregular waves of high frequency and low amplitude.

Table 1: Comparison between rapid eye movement (REM) sleep and non-rapid eye movement (NREM) sleep

	Features	REM sleep	Non REM sleep
1.	Rapid eye movement (REM)	Seen	Not seen
2.	Dreams	Present	Absent

3.	Muscle twitching	Present	Absent
4.	Heart rate	Fluctuating	Stable
5.	Blood pressure	Fluctuating	Stable
6.	Respiration	Fluctuating	Stable
7.	Body temperature	Fluctuating	Stable
8.	Major Neurotransmitter	Noradrenaline	Serotonin

Non-rapid eye movement sleep (NREM or non-REM sleep): Non-rapid eye movement (NREM) is defined as the type of sleep without any movements of eyeballs. It is also known as slow-wave sleep. Dreams never occur in this type of sleep. It occupies almost 70% of total sleeping period. Non-REM sleep is usually followed by REM sleep. The NREM sleep is majorly divided into four stages, based on the EEG pattern. In stage I (also known as stage of drowsiness) alpha waves are gradually diminished and finally abolished. There after it shows low voltage fluctuations with infrequent delta waves. Stage II is the stage of light sleep and characterized by spindle bursts (frequency of 14/ sec), superimposed by low voltage delta waves. In stage III the frequency of delta waves decreases and amplitude increases. In stage IV, delta waves become more prominent with lowest frequency and highest amplitude.

Regulation of sleep: Mammillary body of the posterior hypothalamus is known to be the wake-fullness center of body. Chemical and electrical stimulation of mammillary body leads to wakefulness and its lesion leads to sleep. Onset and maintenance of sleep involves complex pathways between the brain stem reticular formation and cerebral cortex. Raphe nucleus and Locus ceruleus of pons are most important in this aspect.

Major Sleep Disorders

Insomnia: Insomnia is defined as the inability to sleep and abnormal wakefulness. It is the most common type of sleep disorder and usually occurs during systemic illness, mental conditions such as psychiatric problems, alcoholic and drug addiction.

Hypersomnia: Hypersomnia is characterized by an excess need of sleep. It occurs mainly because of lesion in the floor of the third ventricle of brain, formation of brain tumors, chronic bronchitis, encephalitis and disease of muscles. Hypersomnia also occurs in some endocrine disorders such as diabetes insipidus.

Narcolepsy and cataplexy: Narcolepsy is characterized by sudden attack of uncontrollable sleep where cataplexy is sudden outburst of emotion. Both occur due to hypothalamic disorders.

Yoga and sleep: Yoga, a group of physical, mental, and spiritual practices or disciplines, has its own beneficial effect on physical strength and flexibility, breathing, stress and mental focus but the lesser known fact is its positive effects on sleep. A study in 2004 from Harvard Medical School indicates that yoga helps to significantly improve the sleep efficiency, total sleep time, among people suffering from insomnia. Regular practice of asanas like forward bend (Hastapadasana), Cat stretch (Marjariasana), Child pose (Shishuasana), Butterfly pose (Baddha Konasana), Legs-up-the-wall pose (Viparita Karani) gives better sleep at night. 30-90% of cancer survivors suffer from impaired sleep quality post-treatment, which is severe enough to increase morbidity and mortality among the patients. A study conducted in 2013 by Mustian et al. showed the effect of multicenter, randomized controlled trial of yoga for improving sleep quality among cancer survivors. Lymphoma patients also showed improved quality of life after yogic practices. In 2009, silver yoga exercises showed to be beneficial for reducing depression of aged persons.

Yogic Asanas for Better Sleep

Padhastasana

Procedure

1. Bend forward from the hips until the fingers or palms of the hands touch the floor on either side of the feet.
2. Keep the knees straight and bring the forehead as close as possible to the knee.

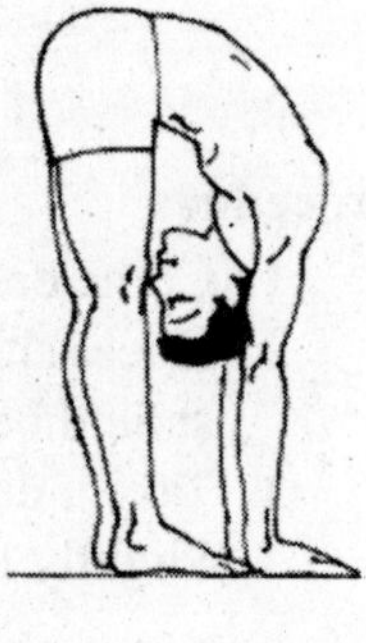

Benefits: Helps stretch the back muscles, invigorates the nervous system by increasing blood supply, and makes the spine supple.

Balasana

Procedure

1. Sit on your heels on a yoga mat or on the floor.
2. Either keep your knees together or apart.
3. Slowly, bend forward by lowering your forehead to touch the floor, exhaling as you do so.
4. Keep your arms alongside your body. Make sure that your palms are facing up.
5. Alternatively, you can reach out your arms towards the front of the yoga mat, palms placed facing down on the mat.
6. Now that you are in this pose, gently press your chest on the thighs (or between the thighs if the latter are apart).
7. Hold for 45 seconds to 1 minute. Regulate your breath.
8. As you inhale, imagine your breath is being driven through your navel, and pull your navel towards your spine.
9. As you exhale, soften your body and the arms. Repeat for 4-12 breaths.
10. Place your palms under the shoulders and gradually raise your upper body to return to the sitting position on the heels while inhaling. Do this very slowly as if uncurling the spine. Relax.

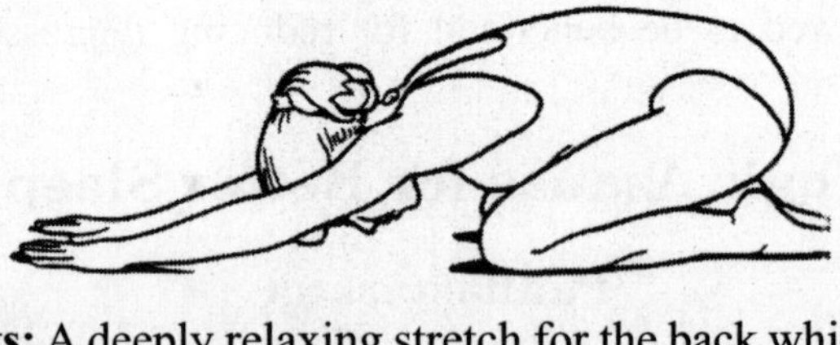

Benefits: A deeply relaxing stretch for the back which also helps calm the nervous system so that you can sleep at peace.

Chakravakasana

Procedure

1. Come onto your hands and knees.
2. Knees should be directly underneath your hips and your hands should be directly underneath your shoulders.
3. Take a deep breath and exhale completely and slowly.
4. Slightly lift your chin.

5. When you inhale, consider that your chest should be expanded and lift it away from your belly.
6. Stretch your front body trunk front by flattening your back.
7. When you stretch your belly in, exhale.
8. Maintain this pose for some minutes.
9. Bring your chest and belly to the thighs and hips to the heels and forehead to the ground after finishing the above pose.
10. Repeat three times at the beginning.
11. Consider about Breathing and maintain a proper time gap.

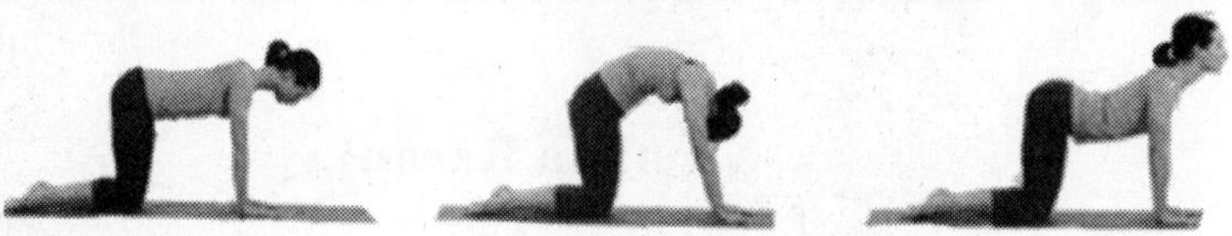

Benefits: Excellent stretch for spine flexibility. Also helps massage the digestive organs and improve digestion, thereby helping you to sleep well. Also improves blood circulation and relaxes the mind.

Badhakonasana

Procedure

1. Sit with your spine erect and legs spread straight out.
2. Now bend your knees and bring your feet towards the pelvis. The soles of your feet should touch each other.
3. Grab your feet tightly with your hands.

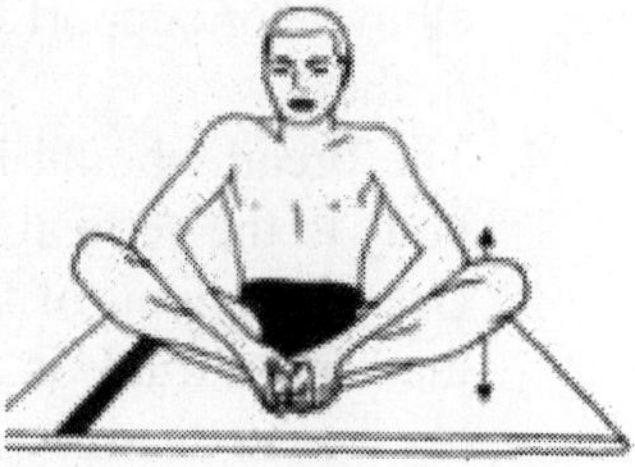

4. Make an effort to bring the heels as close to the genitals as possible.
5. Take a deep breath in. Breathing out, press the thighs and knees downward towards the floor. Make a gentle effort to keep pressing them downward.
6. Now start flapping both the legs up and down like the wings of a butterfly. Start slow and gradually increase the speed. Keep breathing normally throughout.

7. Press your elbows on the thighs or on the knees, pushing the knees and thighs closer to the floor.
8. Feel the stretch in the inner thighs and take long, deep breaths, relaxing the muscles more and more.
9. Take a deep breath in and bring the torso up.
10. As you exhale, gently release the posture. Straighten the legs out in front of you and relax.

Benefits: This pose can help remove fatigue from long hours of standing or walking. Also a good stretch for inner thighs, groin and knees.

Viparita Karani

Procedure

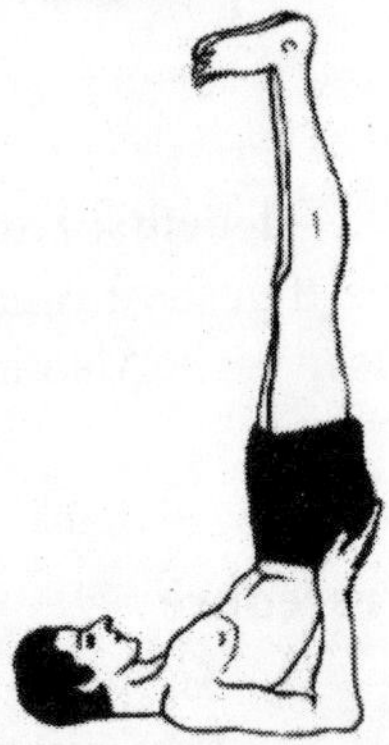

1. Start with the supine position, lying on your back in a relaxed way. Let the hands rest on the floor next to the body and breathe normally.
2. Try to raise the legs slowly till the legs are almost 90 degrees to the floor.
3. Now place the hands under the lower back at the waist level. Use the hands and elbows for support to raise your body up further.
4. The breath should be held inside when you are raising the body to the vertical position.
5. Use the support of the hands to raise the trunk further up, till the whole trunk is about 45 degrees to the ground and the leg are vertical. At this stage the body weight rests on the shoulders. Hands and elbows remain as props to support and balance the body.
6. In the final pose the legs are 90 degrees to the floor and the trunk is about 45 degrees to the floor.
7. Remain in this position according to your comfort. For health benefits 3-5 minutes every day is good enough. Though practitioners can go up to 15 minutes for spiritual benefits.
8. Breathe normally while maintaining the steady raised position.

9. While releasing the position, the breath is held inside and the body is slowly brought down to the supine position.
10. After performing Vipareeta Karani asana, usually a counter asana like Matyasana, Ushtrasana or Supta Vajrasana is performed for half the duration.

Benefits: An excellent pose to relieve tired legs and feet, helps increase blood supply to the brain and relieve mild headache, and calms the mind.

Besides the above, lying down in Shavasana and Yoga Nidra after meals helps relax the entire system.

References

1. Khalsa SB. Treatment of chronic insomnia with yoga: a preliminary study with sleep-wake diaries. Appl Psychophysiol Biofeedback. 2004 Dec; 29(4):269-78.
2. Mustian KM, Sprod LK, Janelsins M, Peppone LJ, Palesh OG, Chandwani K, Reddy PS, Melnik MK, Heckler C, Mor[illegible] GR. Multicenter, randomized controlled trial of yoga for [illegible] quality among cancer survivors. J Clin Oncol. 2013 S[illegible] 31(26):3233-41.
3. Chen KM, Chen MH, Chao HC, Hung HM, Lin HS, [illegible] Sleep quality, depression state, and health status of old adults after silver yoga exercises: cluster randomized trial. [illegible] J Nurs Stud. 2009 Feb; 46(2):154-63.

13
Yoga for Healthy Ageing

In humans, ageing represents the accumulation of changes in human being over the period of time encompassing physical, psychological and social changes. Ageing is gradual continuous process of natural changes that begins in early adulthood, during early middle age, many bodily functions begin to gradually decline.

Cardiovascular diseases are the main killer of older people of both the sexes. With advancing age epicardial fat increases, while the detritus of intracellular catabolism and oxidant stress accumulate in the form of lipofuscin. The size of left ventricular cavity particularly in base to apex dimension is reduced and this volume change is exacerbated by systemic hypertension and bulging of the basal ventricular septum into left ventricular outflow tract. Valvular ageing changes include calcification of the mitral annulus and aortic valve, the latter frequently leading to aortic stenosis. The aorta become progressively stiffer owing to the fragmentation and loss of elastic tissue and increased collagen deposition along with accumulation of atherosclerotic plaque. Compared with younger myocardium elderly myocardium has fewer myocytes, increased collagenised connective tissue and, often deposition and extracellular amyloid (most catabolised transthyretin). Progressive atherosclerosis over a period of 50-60 years finally ends up causing significant stenosis or weakness, the wall sufficiently to give rise to catastrophic dissection of the aortic wall.

Effects of Ageing on Blood Vessels

- Baroreceptors become less sensitive with age. Orthostatic hypotension leads to fall in blood pressure when a person stands from sitting or lying position.

- Capillary walls thicken; lower the exchange of waste and minerals.
- Aorta becomes thicker, blood pressure becomes higher and heart has to work harder, which lead to hypertrophy of heart muscle.

Common Heart Diseases Associated with Ageing

- Angina pectoris
- Anemia
- Coronary artery disease
- Arteriosclerosis
- Arrhythmias
- Congestive heart failure

Prevention

- Reduced cholesterol and saturated fat in the diet.
- Control over blood pressure and weight smoking and alcoholism should be avoided.

Effects of Ageing on Nervous System

- Brain and spinal cord loses nerve cells and weight
- Speed of transmission decreases
- Waste product accumulates in brain and nerve cells
- Slowing of thought, memory and thinking
- Dementia (memory loss)
- Alzheimer disease (due to deposition of lipofuscin).

Prevention

- Exercise keeps blood pressure normal.
- Reading, doing crossword puzzles.

Effects of Ageing on Digestive System

- Digestive system has lot of reserve built into it so, ageing has less effect on its functions compared to other organs.
- With age, strength of oesophageal contraction and tension in upper oesophageal sphincter decreases which make difficulty in swallowing the food.

- As we age, digestive process slows down and causes the food to move slowly through the colon when food moves down, more water get absorbed from food waste which can cause constipation.

Various Diseases of Digestive Systems

1. **Constipation:** Its symptom include; difficult or painful bowel movements, infrequent bowel movements, hard dry stool.
2. **Diverticular disease:** About half of people at 60 or above have diverticulosis. This occurs when small pouches in the lining of the colon bulge out along weak spots in intestinal wall.
3. **Geard** or gastroesophageal reflux disease is the most common upper gastrointestinal disorder in older adults, although of all ages can get it. GEARD occurs when stomach acid backs into oesophagus, causing heartburn.
   Certain medications including some blood pressure medications which many older adults take can cause heartburn. Obesity increases the risk of heartburn and GEARD, so if you gain weight or get older, you could have more reflux.

How to Protect your Digestive Health as you Grow?

1. **Stay active:** Getting at least 30 minutes of exercise 5 days a week can help prevent many age related health problems it will also keep you regular and decrease the risk of colon cancer.
2. **Eat more fiber:** Foods high in fiber including fruits, whole grains and beans tends to be high in nutrients and low in fat.
3. High fiber food can help prevent constipation and ease symptoms of diverticulosis.
4. Drink plenty of fluids throughout the day.

Effects of Ageing on Reproductive System

In females around menopause changes in genital organs occur rapidly. Menstrual cycle stop, ovaries stop producing estrogen.

Unlike women, men do not undergo major rapid change in fertility as they age. Instead changes occur gradually during a process that some people call andropause. Ageing changes in male reproductive system occur primarily in the testis, testicular mass decreases.

Scientific Evidences for Healthy Aging through Yoga

In a cross sectional study, Afonso et al (2017) reported the greater cortical thickness (CT) in elderly female who were pursuing yoga for at least 8 years as compared to control. The authors were found that Yoga practitioners showed significantly greater CT in a left prefrontal lobe cluster, which included portions of the lateral middle frontal gyrus, anterior superior frontal gyrus and dorsal superior frontal gyrus. Eda et al. (2017) found that yoga stretching caused improvement in salivary immune function and mental stress in middle-aged and older adults. Furthermore, the secretary IgA concentration and secretion rate were significantly higher after yoga than before in elderly personnel. Vogler et al. (2011) reported in their study in the journal International Journal of Yoga Therapy, where they found the impact of a short-term Iyengar Yoga program on the health and well-being of physically inactive older adults. The study concluded that participation in Iyengar yoga programs by older people is beneficial for health and well-being, and greater availability of such programs could improve quality of life. Patil et.al (2017) compared yoga and walking-exercise on cardiac time intervals as a measure of cardiac function in elderly with increased pulse pressure. Their study concluded that yoga practice for 3 months showed a significant improvement in diastolic function with a minimal change in systolic function. Yoga is more effective than walking in improving cardiac function in elderly with high pulse pressure. Lelard et al. (2017) reported that during gait initiation, postural adjustments are needed to deal with balance and movement. With aging, gait initiation changes and reflects functional degradation of frailty in individuals. However, physical activities have demonstrated beneficial effects of daily motor tasks. The authors reported that yoga practitioners had slower center of pressure displacements and lower leg muscles % of co-activation in comparison with walkers. Hunter et al. (2017) studied the effect of Bikram yoga on endothelial function in young and middle-aged and older adults. The results demonstrated that a relatively short-term Bikram yoga practice significantly improve vascular endothelial function in middle-aged and older adults. While apparently healthy individuals in this study experienced no adverse events, those with pre-existing conditions should take caution and consult with a physician prior to engaging in this style of yoga. A randomized controlled trial of Kundalini yoga on elderly personnel were reported by Eyre et al. (2017), they found that Kundalini yoga group showed short and long-term improvements in executive functioning as compared to memory enhancement training, and broader effects on depressed mood and resilience. In conclusion, regular practice of yoga asanas, pranayama and meditation can lead to a happier and more fulfilling life. Yoga will not just tone your body, but will also uplift your mind. Your attitude will improve. You will think and feel young.

As age progresses, it is important to focus on how you do yoga rather than how much you do. Here some yoga modules are described which will be useful for elderly personnel.

(A) Standing Yoga Asanas

1. Trikonasana

Procedure

1. Stand erect and keep distance between your legs about 3 to 4 feet.
2. Extend your arms at the shoulder level.
3. Inhale and raise your right arm by the side of your head.
4. Now, bend your right arms with exhaling towards the left side by keeping your body weight equally on both the feet. You should ensure that the right arm become parallel to the ground.
5. Maintain the position as per your comfort with normal breathing (for 5-10 seconds) and come to the original position by inhaling.
6. Do the same procedure with the left arm.

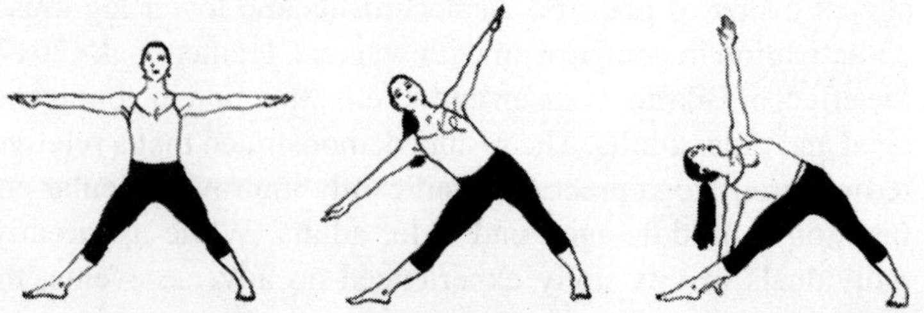

Benefits: Hip problems are routine among seniors. Trikonasana helps strengthen and stretch the hip region. It helps regulate blood pressure, a common complaint amongst the elderly.

2. Katichakrasana

Procedure

1. Stand up straight with your feet together.
2. As you breathe in, stretch your hands to the front, palms facing each other, parallel to the ground.
3. Exhale and gently twist from the waist to the right and look back over the right shoulder.
4. Keep the distance between your palms constant.
5. Breathing in, come back to the center.
6. Breathing out, turn to your left and repeat the yoga posture on your left side.
7. Breathing in, come back to the center.
8. Repeat this yoga pose a few times on both sides and then breathing out, bring your hands down.

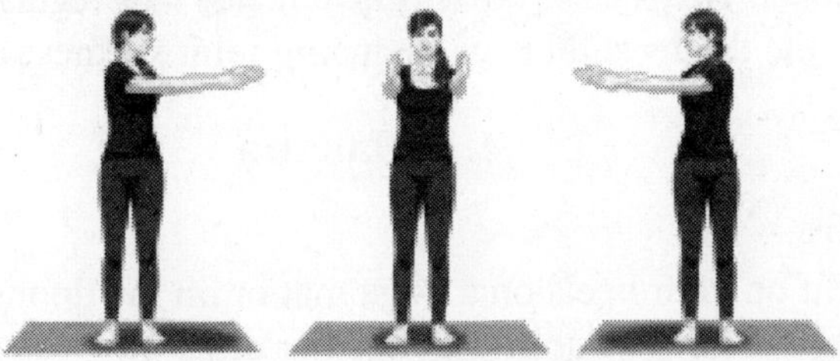

Benefits: It helps to keep the spine straight; helps strengthen the arm and leg muscles.

(B) Sitting Yoga Asana

3. Badhakonasana

Procedure

1. Sit with your spine erect and legs spread straight out.
2. Now bend your knees and bring your feet towards the pelvis. The soles of your feet should touch each other.
3. Grab your feet tightly with your hands.

4. Make an effort to bring the heels as close to the genitals as possible.
5. Take a deep breath in. Breathing out, press the thighs and knees downward towards the floor. Make a gentle effort to keep pressing them downward.

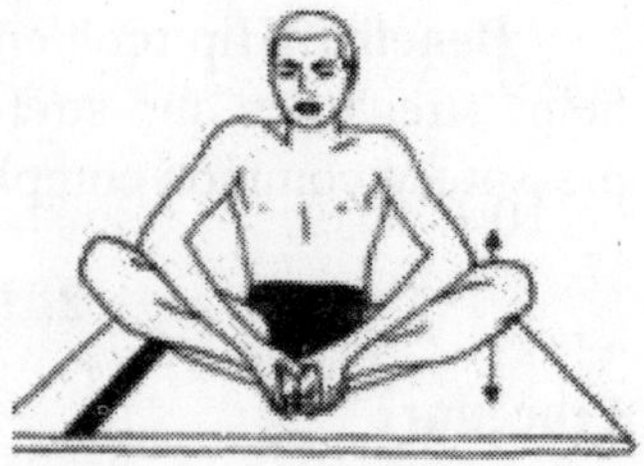

6. Now start flapping both the legs up and down like the wings of a butterfly. Start slow and gradually increase the speed. Keep breathing normally throughout.
7. Press your elbows on the thighs or on the knees, pushing the knees and thighs closer to the floor.
8. Feel the stretch in the inner thighs and take long, deep breaths, relaxing the muscles more and more.
9. Take a deep breath in and bring the torso up.
10. As you exhale, gently release the posture. Straighten the legs out in front of you and relax.

Benefits: Helps clear bowel movements, thus regulating digestion. Stretches the thighs and knees, reducing joint stiffness and pain.

4. Balasana

Procedure

1. Sit on your heels on a yoga mat or on the floor.
2. Either keep your knees together or apart.
3. Slowly, bend forward by lowering your forehead to touch the floor, exhaling as you do so.
4. Keep your arms alongside your body. Make sure that your palms are facing up.
5. Alternatively, you can reach out your arms towards the front of the yoga mat, palms placed facing down on the mat.
6. Now that you are in this pose, gently press your chest on the thighs (or between the thighs if the latter are apart).
7. Hold for 45 seconds to 1 minute. Regulate your breath.
8. As you inhale, imagine your breath is being driven through your navel, and pull your navel towards your spine.

9. As you exhale, soften your body and the arms. Repeat for 4-12 breaths.
10. Place your palms under the shoulders and gradually raise your upper body to return to the sitting position on the heels while inhaling. Do this very slowly as if uncurling the spine. Relax.

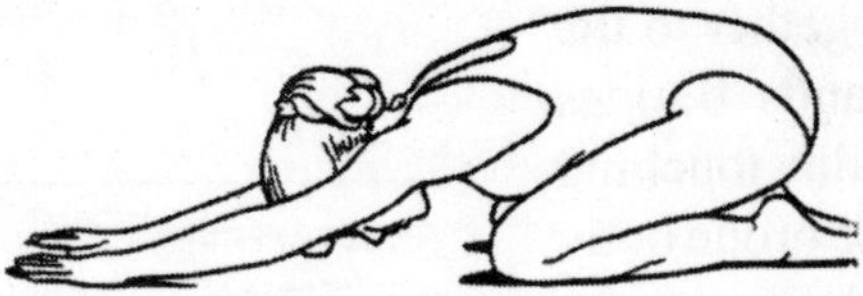

Benefits: It eases anxiety and stress. Focusing on the breathing helps relax the mind. It is beneficial in neurocognition.

5. Chakravakasana

Procedure

1. Come onto your hands and knees.
2. Knees should be directly underneath your hips and your hands should be directly underneath your shoulders.
3. Take a deep breath and exhale completely and slowly.
4. Slightly lift your chin.
5. When you inhale, consider that your chest should be expanded and lift it away from your belly.
6. Stretch your front body trunk front by flattening your back.
7. When you stretch your belly in, exhale.
8. Maintain this pose for some minutes.
9. Bring your chest and belly to the thighs and hips to the heels and forehead to the ground after finishing the above pose.
10. Repeat three times at the beginning.
11. Contemplate about the breathing and maintain a proper time gap.

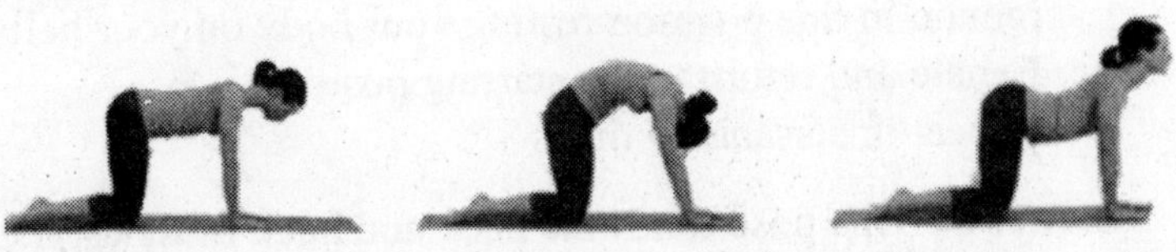

Benefits: It helps to easing the stress in the low back and gives the normal breathing flow and peace of mind. One can feel the calmness and the peace of mind. It is beneficial in neurocognition.

(C) Yoga poses lying on the back or stomach

6. Bhujangasana

Procedure

Lie down on abdomen with legs close together to the ground. Place hands besides the body with palm touching on ground. Lift the prone body from the ground up to the naval region.

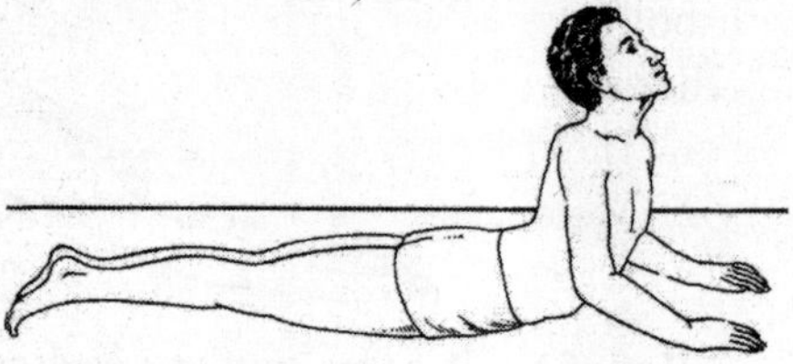

Maintain the position for 5-10 seconds or as long as comfortable.

Benefits: Improves blood circulation that weakens with age. It strengthens the back and shoulders.

7. Shalabhasana

Procedure

1. Lie down on the floor on your belly and place your chin on the floor.
2. Place your toes on the floor; touch the knees to the ground.
3. Place your hands below the hips on the ground below your hips in a way that your palms rest on the ground.
4. While inhaling lift up your head, upper body, thighs and legs off the floor.

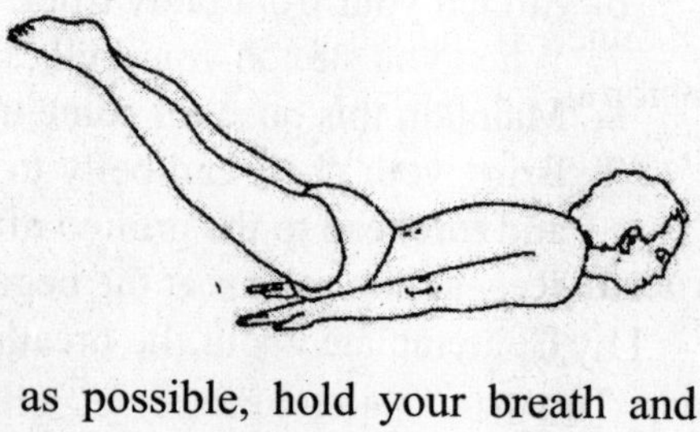

5. Raise your leg as high as possible, hold your breath and remain in this position resting your body on your belly.
6. Exhale and return to the starting position.
7. Repeat this asana 10 times.

Benefits: This pose tones the neck and back muscles, increasing flexibility. It also tones the abdominal organs, improving digestion.

8. Pawanmuktasana

Procedure

It relieves pain and strengthens musculoskeletal system. It is performed first with the right lower limb, then with the left and then with both the lower limbs together. Lie on your back with your feet together and arms beside your body.

1. Lie down on your back and extend the legs and arms.
2. With each exhale, draw both of your knees to your chest. Clasp your hands around your knees.
3. While holding only your right knee, release your left leg and extend it along the floor. Hold this pose for 30 seconds to 1 minute.

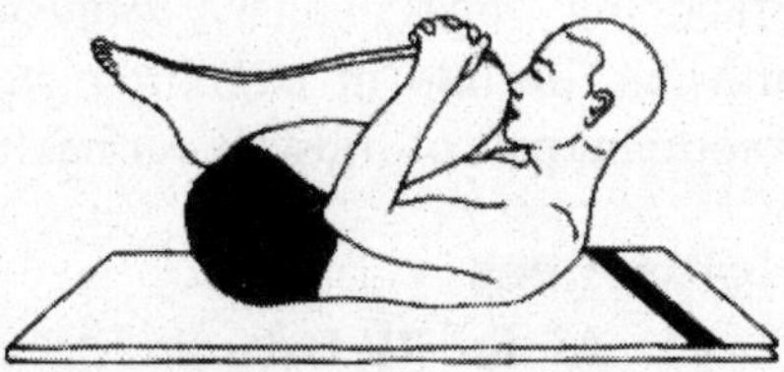

4. Draw your left knee back in towards your chest and clasp your hands around both knees again.
5. While holding only your left knee, release your right leg and extend it along the floor. Hold this pose for the same amount of time.
6. Finally, draw both knees to your chest.

Benefits: Releases flatulence, a common digestive issue in elderly personnel. It increases blood circulation to the hip joints, releasing tension in the area.

9. Savasana

Procedure

Lay down on your back allow your arms and legs to relax by your sides. Turn your palms up. Close your eyes and breathe slowly and deeply. When you are settled, begin to mentally observe and release any tension in your body.

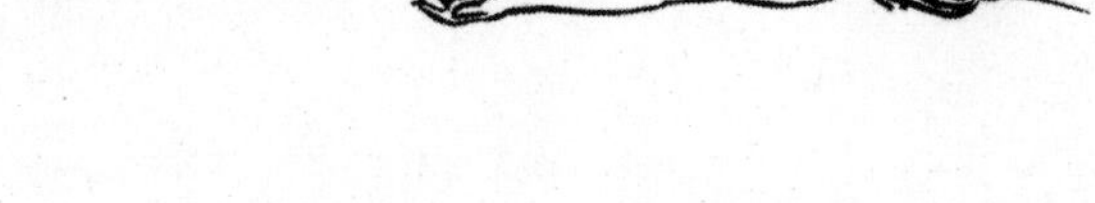

Benefits: Savasana relaxes whole body, relieves physical and mental fatigue. Extremely beneficial for high blood pressure and relieving stress.

Pranayamas

Anulom Vilom- 10 min

Followed by Om chanting for 10 min

In summary, over time, as the age increases there is loss of cartilage, and the joint spacing between bones can become smaller. Practicing yoga regularly prevents age related problems such as arthritis, decline in cognition etc. Consider the yogic regimen as important part of lifestyle for healthy ageing.

References

1. Afonso RF, Balardin JB, Lazar S, Sato JR, Igarashi N, Santaella DF, Lacerda SS, Amaro E Jr, Kozasa EH. Greater Cortical Thickness in Elderly Female Yoga Practitioners-A Cross-Sectional Study. Front Aging Neurosci. 2017 Jun 20;9:201.
2. Vogler J, O'Hara L, Gregg J, Burnell F. The impact of a short-term iyengar yoga program on the health and well-being of physically inactive older adults. Int J Yoga Therap. 2011;(21):61-72.
3. Eda N, Ito H, Shimizu K, Suzuki S, Lee E, Akama T. Yoga stretching for improving salivary immune function and mental stress in middle-aged and older adults. J Women Aging. 2017 Apr 3:1-15.
4. Hunter SD, Dhindsa MS, Cunningham E, Tarumi T, Alkatan M, Nualnim N, Elmenshawy A, Tanaka H. The effect of Bikram yoga on endothelial function in young and middle-aged and older adults. J Bodyw Mov Ther. 2017 Jan;21(1):30-34.
5. Eyre HA, Siddarth P, Acevedo B, Van Dyk K, Paholpak P, Ercoli L, St Cyr N, Yang H, Khalsa DS, Lavretsky H. A randomized controlled trial of Kundalini yoga in mild cognitive impairment. Int Psychogeriatr. 2017 Apr; 29(4):557-567.

❐

14
Yoga for Prevention of Cardiovascular Diseases

Cardiovascular diseases (CVDs) are caused when the problems arise in the heart and blood vessels, and include heart attacks, stroke, hypertension, peripheral artery disease, rheumatic heart disease, congenital heart disease and heart failure. The major causes of cardiovascular disease are tobacco use, physical inactivity, an unhealthy diet and harmful use of alcohol. According to world health organization, 17.5 million people die every year from CVDs, an estimated 31% of all deaths worldwide. It is found that more than 75% of CVD deaths occur in low-income and middle-income countries while 80% of all CVD deaths are due to heart attacks and strokes.

Overview of CVDs

1. Coronary Heart Disease: When flow of oxygen-rich blood to a section of heart muscle suddenly blocked and the heart cannot get oxygen then it results in heart attack. If the oxygenated blood does not restore, the heart muscles begin to die. It occurs when cholesterol accumulation leads to formation of plaques in the coronary artery, which stops the blood flow to the heart.

2. Cerebrovascular Disease: Cerebrovascular disease or stroke happens when a blood vessel that carries oxygen to the brain gets blocked or bursts and blood cannot deliver oxygen to part of the brain and that part of the brain starts to die. Without the right medical attention, a stroke can cause major damage to the brain. A person with attack of stroke may have problems in speaking, seeing or moving normally for a short time or for the rest of their lives. The person can even die from a stroke. Older adults are more likely to have a stroke than younger people, but people can have a stroke at any age. Other factors that increase risk of stroke include high blood pressure, cigarette smoking, diabetes, other types of cardiovascular disease, and high blood cholesterol.

3. Hypertension: High blood pressure or hypertension is an important risk factor for heart disease, and many people do not have any symptoms when their blood pressure is high. People with high blood pressure are more likely to have a heart attack or stroke than people with normal blood pressure.

You can control your blood pressure by adopting following healthy habits:

a. Keep your weight healthy.
b. Eat a heart-healthy diet with lower levels of sodium.
c. Getting enough regular physical activity.

4. Peripheral Artery Disease: Peripheral artery disease is a disease in which plaque builds up in the arteries that carry blood to brain, organs, and limbs. Plaque is made up of fat, cholesterol, calcium, fibrous tissue, and other substances in the blood. When plaque builds up in the body's arteries, the condition is called atherosclerosis. Over time, plaque can harden and narrow the arteries. This limits the flow of oxygen-rich blood to your organs and other parts of your body. It affects the arteries in the legs, but it also can affect the arteries that carry blood from heart to head, arms, kidneys, and stomach.

5. Rheumatic Heart Disease: Rheumatic heart disease damage to one or more heart valves that remains after an episode of acute rheumatic fever is resolved. It is caused by an episode or recurrent episodes of acute rheumatic fever, where the heart has become inflamed. The heart valves can remain stretched and/or scarred, and normal blood flow through damaged valves is interrupted. Blood may flow backward through stretched valves that do not close properly, or may be blocked due to scarred valves not opening properly. When the heart is damaged in this way, the heart valves are unable to function adequately, and heart surgery may be required. Untreated, rheumatic heart disease causes heart failure and those affected are at risk of arrhythmias, stroke, endocarditis and complications of pregnancy. These conditions cause progressive disability, reduce quality of life and can cause premature death in young adults. Heart surgery can manage some of these problems and prolong life but does not cure Rheumatic heart disease.

6. Congenital Heart Disease: A congenital heart disease is a problem with heart's structure that is there when a baby is born. It happens by incomplete or abnormal development of the fetus's heart during the very early weeks of pregnancy. The cause of most congenital heart defects is unknown. Though, they cannot be prevented, there are many treatments for the defects and related health problems.

Functioning of Heart

The human body consist of different systems. Heart lung and blood vessels make up the circulatory system. The heart is the central pump of circulatory system, and consists of four chambers: the left atrium and left ventricle and the right atrium and right ventricle. The heart also has four valves that direct the flow of blood through the heart:

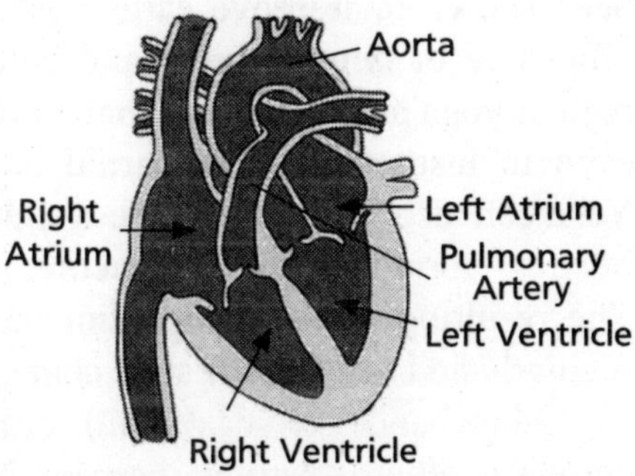

- The left atrium of the heart receives oxygen-rich blood from the lungs and then empties into the left ventricle through the mitral valve.
- The left ventricle pumps oxygen-rich blood out to the rest of the body. Blood leaves the left ventricle through the aortic valve and enters the aorta, the largest artery in the body. Blood then flows from the aorta into the branches of many smaller arteries, providing the body's organs and tissues with the oxygen and nutrients they need.
- After oxygen in the blood is released to the tissues, the now deoxygenated blood returns to the heart through veins, the blood vessels that carry deoxygenated blood. This blood, which looks blue, enters the right atrium of the heart and then travels across the tricuspid valve into the right ventricle.
- The right ventricle then pumps deoxygenated blood through the pulmonic valve into the lungs. The oxygen in the air we breathe binds to cells within this blood that is being pumped through the lungs. The oxygen-rich blood, which appears red, then returns to the left atrium and enters the left ventricle, where it is pumped out to the body once again.

This is the normal circulatory pathway by which blood travels through the heart and the body.

Scientific Evidences of Yoga for betterment of Heart Diseases

Yoga as a form of physical exercise, if done vigorously can raise the heart rate into the aerobic range, potentially lowering the risk of a future heart attack. Even pranayama (yogic breathing) alone has been shown to improve cardiovascular conditioning. The improved efficiency of lung function and better oxygenation that comes with regular yoga practice means that more oxygen reaches the heart muscle even in instances where partial blockage compromise blood flow. Yoga can also lead to decrease weight and stress hormones. Lowering of stress hormones lessens appetite. Doing yoga makes you feel better. The resulting increase in optimism can encourage practicing yoga regularly and making life style changes that contribute to better health.

Manchanda et al. (2003) evaluated yoga, on retardation of coronary atherosclerotic disease. In this prospective, randomized, controlled trial, 42 men with angiographically proven CAD were randomized to control (n = 21) and yoga intervention group (n = 21) and were followed for 1 year. The active group was treated with a user-friendly program consisting of yoga, control of risk factors, diet control and moderate aerobic exercise. The control group was managed by conventional methods i.e. risk factor control and American Heart Association step I diet. At 1 year, the yoga groups showed significant reduction in number of anginal episodes per week, improved exercise capacity and decrease in body weight. Serum total cholesterol, LDL cholesterol and triglyceride levels also showed greater reductions as compared with control group. Revascularisation procedures (coronary angioplasty or bypass surgery) were less frequently required in the yoga group. Coronary angiography repeated at 1 year showed that significantly more lesions regressed (20% versus 2%) and less lesions progressed (5% versus 37%) in the yoga group (chi-square = 24.9; $P < 0.0001$). The compliance of the total program was excellent and no side effects were observed. Authors were concluded that yoga lifestyle intervention retards progression and increases regression of coronary atherosclerosis in patients with severe coronary artery disease. Yogendra et. al (2004) in a small prospective, controlled, open trial evaluated yoga based lifestyle modifications help in regression of coronary lesions and in improving myocardial perfusion. The study concluded that yoga based intervention is translated into clinical benefits and symptomatic improvement. Furthermore, Pullen et al. (2008) reported the effects of yoga on inflammation and exercise capacity in patients with chronic heart failure. They hypothesized that an 8-week regimen of yoga in addition to standard medical therapy would improve exercise capacity, inflammatory markers, and quality of life in patients with heart failure. A total of 19 patients were enrolled after the initial screening and study concluded that Yoga improved exercise tolerance and positively affected levels of inflammatory markers in patients with heart failure, and there was also a trend toward improvements in quality of life. In another study Hagins et al. (2013) reported the Effectiveness of Yoga for Hypertension in a Systematic Review and Meta-Analysis. The result obtained was concluded that Yoga can be preliminarily recommended as an effective intervention for reducing blood pressure. Hari Krishna et. al (2014) studied 130 randomly selected heart failure patients in two groups. Twelve week yoga therapy significantly improved the parasympathetic activity and decreased the sympathetic activity in heart failure patients. In another study, Raghuram et. al (2014) compared the long term effects of yoga based cardiac rehabilitation program with only physiotherapy based program as an add-on to conventional rehabilitation after coronary artery pass grafting on risk factors in 250 males. The yoga group had significantly better improvement in left ventricular ejection fraction (LVEF) than control group in those with abnormal baseline EF after 1 year. There was a better reduction in BMI in the yoga group in those with high baseline BMI after 12 months. A study published in the European Journal of Preventive Cardiology (Chu *et al.,* 2016) found that practicing yoga had the same effect on reducing cardiovascular markers as other forms of exercise, like brisk walking. The researchers reviewed 37 earlier studies that included almost 2800 people. The participants were randomly assigned to do yoga or "regular" exercise like biking and walking; a control group consisted of those who were not asked to add anything to their routine. The participants' yoga practices averaged about 12 weeks, but were as short as three and as long as 52. Yoga and other forms of exercise both had favourable effects on several measures of heart and metabolic health. Body mass index (BMI) was reduced, low-density (bad) cholesterol was reduced by 12 mg/dl, and high-density (good) cholesterol rose by 3 mg/dl. Blood pressure and heart rate also dropped, as did total cholesterol.

In summary, yoga is useful in primary and secondary prevention of CVD but there are several limitations of the reported studies. Most of the studies have small sample size and have inconsistencies in baseline; many studies have absence of adequate controls and have non-uniform methodologies.

Yogic regimen for prevention of CVD (Adapted from published reports)

Asana, pranayam and meditation are the key yogic regimen for prevention of heart diseases.

Asanas

1. Neck Movement: Sit in a comfortable position with your back straight but not rigid. Close your eyes. Bring awareness to the breath, and observe it as it flows in and out, gently and through your nose. Now you are ready to begin the neck movements:

Procedure

- Keep your spinal cord and neck straight.
- Close your eyes and keep both the palms on your knees.
- Concentrate on your neck.
- Now inhale deep and move your neck backward as much as you can but do not strain.
- Remain in the same position for 2-3 seconds and feel the tensioning in the muscle.
- Now move the neck downward and try to touch the collarbone with your chin.
- Exhale completely while bringing the neck downward.
- This is the first cycle of the exercise.
- Repeat this exercise for 10-15 times.

Breathing Pattern

- Inhale while moving the neck backward.
- Exhale while moving the neck downward.

2. Shoulder Movement: Sit in a comfortable position with your arm loose at your sides. Practice the following shoulder movements:

- Inhale and raise your shoulders up towards the ears.

- Exhale and move your shoulders forward and toward each other.
- Inhale and bring your shoulders down.
- Exhale and bring your shoulders back, moving the shoulder blades together.
- Repeat above steps for several cycles.

3. Ankle Movement: Sit on the floor with your legs stretched out in front of you. Practice the following ankle movements:

- Exhale and point your toes away from you. Inhale and lift your toes toward you. Repeat twice more.
- Move your toes in a clockwise direction, keeping your legs still so the movement comes from your ankles, not your legs. Begin slowly at first, then increase the size of the circle and the speed. Do it three more times. Repeat in the opposite direction.

4. Knee to chest pose

Procedure

1. From lying on the floor, bring your knees to your chest and wrap your arms around your legs, giving yourself a big hug.
2. Inhale, and roll your shoulders down, away from the ears and underneath you, opening the heart.
3. Exhale as you use the strength of your arms to squeeze and gently press the thighs down towards the core. Slight tuck the chin to elongate the top of the spine on the neck.
4. Go through steps 2 and 3 for as long as you want to stay here. Just gently release the legs and lay down in Savasana.

5. Relaxation poses (Savasana) for 1 minute: Lay down on your back allow your arms and legs to relax by your sides. Turn your palms up. Close your eyes and breathe slowly and deeply. When you are settled, begin to mentally observe and release any tension in your body. Savasana, relaxes whole body, relieves physical and mental fatigue. Extremely beneficial for high blood pressure and relieving stress.

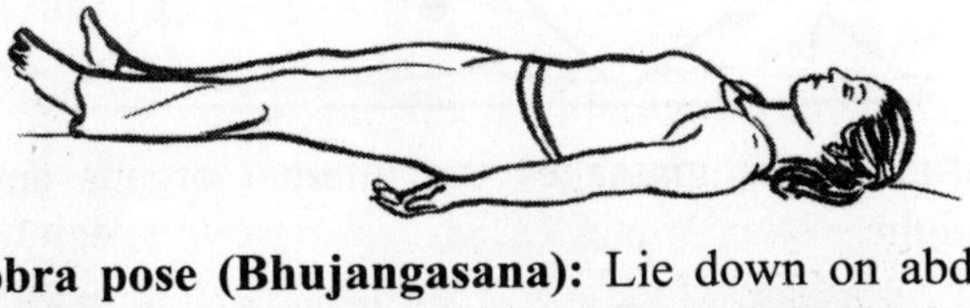

6. Cobra pose (Bhujangasana): Lie down on abdomen with legs close together to the ground. Place hands besides the body with palm touching on ground. Lift the prone body from the ground up to the naval region.

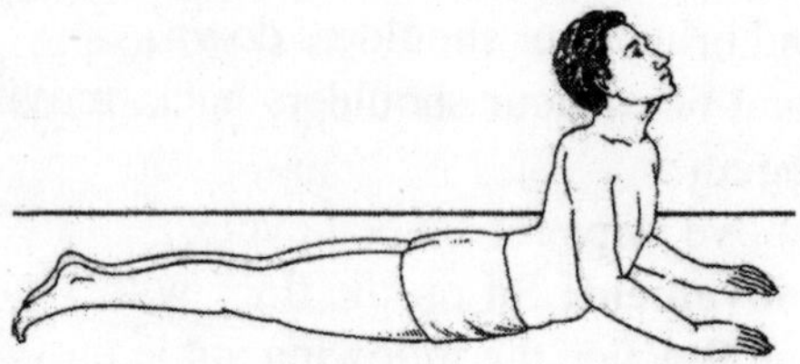

Maintain the position for 5 -10 seconds or as long as comfortable. This asanarelieves in improving lung and heart function.

7. Salabhasana: Lie down on the floor on your belly and place your chin on the floor. Place your toes on the floor, touch the knees to the ground. Place your hands below the hips on the ground below your hips in a way that your palms rest on the ground. While inhaling lift up your head, upper body, thighs and legs off the floor. Raise your leg as high as possible, hold your breath and remain in this position resting your body on your belly. Exhale and return to the starting position. It helps in relieving you of stress and calms your mind, body and soul and is beneficial for depression.

8. Savasana (for one minute): Repeat as described above

9. Paschimottanasana: Sit on the floor with the legs outstretched, feet together and hands on the knees. Slowly bend forward from the hips, sliding the hands down the legs. Try to grasp the big toes with the fingers and thumbs. Move slowly without forcing or jerking. Hold the position for a few seconds. Relax the back and leg muscles, allowing them to gently stretch. Keeping the legs straight and utilizing the arm muscles, not the back muscles, begin to bend the elbows and gently bring the trunk down towards the legs, maintaining a firm grip on the toes, feet or legs. Try to touch the knees with the forehead.

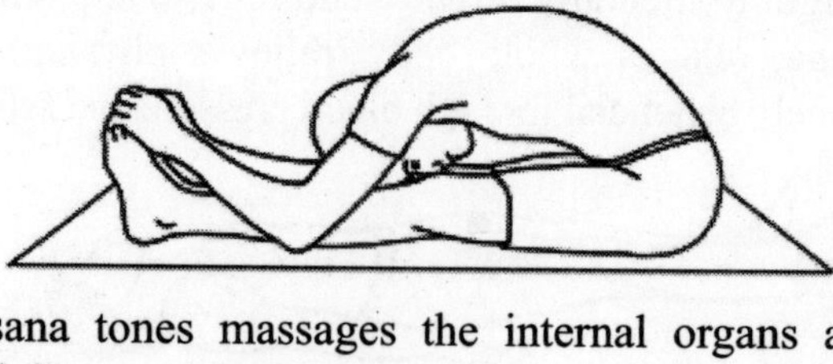

This asana tones massages the internal organs and helps to maintain weight.

10. Savasana (for one minute): Repeat as described above.

11. Salamba Sarvangasana: Lie on your back near a wall, with your knees bent and your buttocks as close to the wall as possible. Turn your palms down and press them into the floor. Bring the soles of your feet to the wall, and begin to walk up the wall. As you do this, bring your hand to your lower back for support. Breathe normally and go up only as high as is comfortable, without any strain. If you are comfortable doing so, straighten your legs, allowing them to lean against the wall. If you develop dizziness or feel pressure in your head or neck, come out of the pose right away. Otherwise stay up for one minute or less, and gradually build up your time in this pose to 2-3 minutes. Come out of the pose slowly by walking your feet down the wall and lowering your buttocks to the floor.

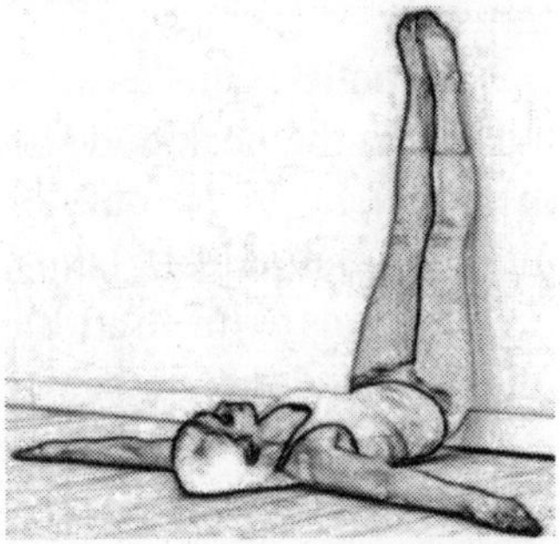

Benefits: This asana Stretches the shoulders and neck; tones the legs, buttocks, and abdomen, regulates metabolism digestion; calms the brain and helps to relieve stress and mild depression; help to reduce weight; reduces fatigue and alleviates insomnia and helps to reduce varicose veins.

12. Savasana (for one minute): Repeat as described above

13. Matsyasana: Lie on your back. Your feet are together and hands relaxed alongside the body. Place the hands underneath the hips, palms facing down. Bring the elbows closer toward each other. Breathing in, lift the head and chest up. Keeping the chest elevated, lower the head backward and touch the top of the head to the floor. With the head lightly touching the floor, press the elbows firmly into the ground, placing the weight on the elbow and not on the head. Lift your chest up from in-between the shoulder blades. Press the thighs and legs to the floor. Hold the pose for as long as you comfortably can, taking gentle long breaths in and out. Relax in the posture with every exhalation. Now lift the head up, lowering the chest and head to the floor. Bring the hands back along the sides of the body. Relax.

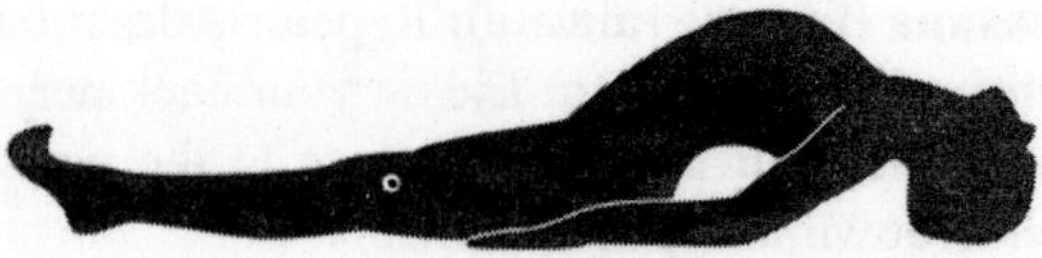

Benefits: This asana stretches the chest and neck. It helps relieve tension in the neck and shoulders and provides relief from respiratory disorders by encouraging deep breathing. It tones the parathyroid, pituitary and pineal glands. This pose is beneficial to prevent CVDs.

Persons with high blood pressure, lower-back or neck injuries, migraine and insomnia should not practice this pose.

14. Savasana (for one minute): Repeat as described above

15. Ardhmatsyendrasan: Sit in Vajrasana position or sit straight by stretching your legs in front of you. Bend your left leg and try to touch your feet to your right buttock as shown in the image. Bring your right leg outside of the left knee. Touch your feet to the ground. Keep your spine erect. Exhale and turn your upper body to the right. Hold your right feet with left hand and place your right hand behind you are on the ground as shown in the above image. Breathe normally and hold this posture for 20 to 30 seconds. After practicing you can hold this posture for 2 to 3 minutes or as you feel comfortable. Now release this posture and repeat this cycle with bending right leg and bringing left leg outside of the right knee. (i.e. Twisting the opposite direction).

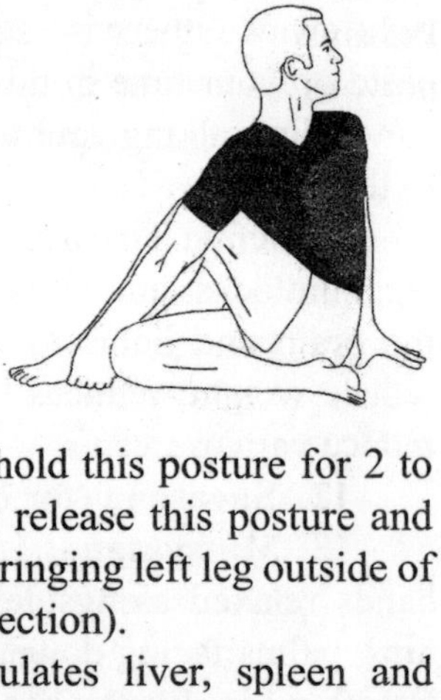

Benefits: It relieves back pain, stimulates liver, spleen and pancreas and helps to regulate their functioning and benefits intestines also. It also strengthens the spinal column and muscles of the back. Beneficial in prevention of CVDs.

16. Yog mudra: Perform it for 30-60 seconds. Sit in a comfortable cross legged position with your eyes closed. Bring your arms behind your back and take hold of your right wrist. Inhale and stretch your arms up. Exhale, extend your chin, and fold your body forward over your legs. When you have come forward as much as you comfortably can, allow your body and head to relax. To come out of the pose, inhale, extend your chin, and slowly raise your head and body back to a seated position. As you exhale, bring your palms together at the chest, and feel the effects of yog mudra.

17. Savasana (for one minute): Repeat as described above

18. Pranyam Nadi shodhan: Sit relaxed and concentrate on the normal breath for a few minutes. Lift the right hand, place the index finger and middle finger at the centre of the eyebrows(Pranayama Mudra) and close the right nostril with the thumb. Breathe through the left nostril 20 times - the breath should be slightly deeper than normal and directed into the abdomen. Open the right nostril again and close the left nostril with the ring finger. Breathe through the right nostril 20 times - the breath is slightly deeper than normal and into the abdomen. Return the hand to the knee and observe the normal flow of the breath.

Benefits: Nadi Shodhana purifies the blood and respiratory system. The deeper breathing enriches the blood with oxygen. This Pranayama strengthens the respiratory system and balances the nervous system. It helps to relieve nervousness and headaches.

19. Meditation: Comfortably sit on the floor and close your eyes. During the silence, concentrate the mind on one thing. Just focus on peace and stillness within. Check your posture and keep your body still during this entire time. As body becomes still and quiet, the mind follows. Stay for a minute or longer, building up gradually over time.

References

1. Pullen PR, Nagamia SH, Mehta PK, Thompson WR, Benardot D, Hammoud R, Parrott JM, Sola S, Khan BV. Effects of yoga on inflammation and exercise capacity in patients with chronic heart failure. J Card Fail. 2008 Jun; 14(5):407-13.
2. Chu P, Gotink RA, Yeh GY, Goldie SJ, Hunink MG. The effectiveness of yoga in modifying risk factors for cardiovascular disease and metabolic syndrome: A systematic review and meta-analysis of randomized controlled trials. Eur J Prev Cardiol. 2016 Feb; 23(3):291-307.
3. Manchanda SC, Narang R, Reddy KS, Sachdeva U, Prabhakaran D, Dharmanand S, Rajani M, Bijlani R. Reversal of coronary atherosclerosis by yoga lifestyle intervention. In Frontiers in Cardiovascular Health 2003 (pp. 535-547). Springer US.

4. Hagins M, Selfe T, Innes K. Effectiveness of yoga for hypertension: systematic review and meta-analysis. Evidence-Based Complementary and Alternative Medicine. 2013 May 28; 2013.
5. Hari Krishna et.al Effect of yoga therapy on heart rate, blood pressure and cardiac autonomic function in heart failure. Journal of clinical and diagnostic research. 2014, 8 (1): 14-16.
6. Raghuram et al. 2014. Yoga based cardiac rehabilitation after coronary artery bypass surgery: One year results on LVEF, lipid profile and psychological states-A randomized controlled study. Indian heart journal. 2014, 66: 490-502.
7. Yogendra J, Yogendra HJ, Ambardekar S, Lele RD, Shetty S, Dave M, Husein N. Beneficial effects of yoga lifestyle on reversibility of ischaemic heart disease: caring heart project of International Board of Yoga. J Assoc Physicians India. 2004 Apr; 52:283-9.
8. McCall T. Yoga as medicine: The yogic prescription for health and healing. Bantam; 2007 Jul 31.

Note: Images shown for understanding of asanas; Source: Google

❑

15
Yoga for Prevention of Diabetes

Diabetes is a common condition in which the amount of glucose in the blood is too high because the body is unable to use it properly. It can occur at any age but incidence increases with age. The hormone secreted by Pancreas, known as insulin controls the amount of glucose in the blood.

In 2014, 8.5% of adults aged 18 years and older had diabetes. In 2012, diabetes was the direct cause of 1.5 million deaths and high blood glucose was the cause of another 2.2 million deaths (WHO).

Food and Insulin

Food is taken in and travels through the gut. The pancreas secretes insulin when we eat and food is broken into smaller molecules such as glucose in the gut. After a meal, blood glucose levels rise and insulin is normally released into the blood. Insulin is crucial to stop blood glucose levels rising too high. Diabetes develops when the pancreas is unable to produce insulin or when cells cannot use the insulin properly.

Types of Diabetes

Type 1 diabetes develops when there is a severe lack of insulin in the body because most or all insulin producing beta cells in the pancreas have been destroyed. This is treated by insulin injections and diet. It is an auto-immune disorder.

Type 2 diabetes develops when pancreas still produces insulin but there is cellular resistance and insulin cannot be used properly by the body. This is treated by diet alone or diet and tablets, or diet and insulin injections. It is known as diabetes mellitus. It occurs by metabolic disorders.

Table 1: Difference between type-I and type-II diabetes

	Type-I Diabetes	Type-II Diabetes
Age of onset	Young < 40yr	Older > 40yr
Symptoms	Yes-very sudden/intense	Sometimes-slow gradual onset
Auto immune	Yes	No
Producing own insulin	No	Yes
Body Weight	Normal	Normal/overweight
Treatment	Insulin	Diet/tablets/Insulin

Hypoglycaemia (Blood glucose below 4 mmol/l or 72 mg/dL) signs and symptoms: If glucose levels become too low, as occurs with hypoglycemia, it can cause these signs and symptoms:

- Sweating: Excessive sweating can be a warning sign of diabetes.
- Shaking
- Headaches
- Blurred vision
- Dizziness
- Tingling lips/fingers/tongue
- Palpitations
- Feeling hungry
- Lack of concentration
- Pallor
- Glazed eyes
- Personality changes/behavioural changes

Many conditions other than hypoglycemia may cause these signs and symptoms. But to be sure that these symptoms are due to hypoglycemia require blood sugar test to know for sure that hypoglycemia is the cause.

Hyperglycaemia signs and symptoms: If a person with a consistent range above 7 mol/l or 126 mg/dl is generally held to have hyperglycemia, he/she may have following symptoms

a) Thirst

b) Tiredness
c) Polyuria (frequency passing urine particularly at night)
d) Weight loss
e) Fast breathing
f) Vomiting – late stages
g) Impaired consciousness
h) Increased risk of infections (in particular thrush)

Complications of Diabetes

Eye damage

a) Diabetic Retinopathy (bleeding at the back of the eye & formation of new vessels)
b) If untreated can lead to blindness.
c) People with diabetes need to have annual screening for early signs of eye damage

Kidney damage

a) Diabetic Nephropathy is the formation of small new blood vessels in the kidneys, if undetected can lead to renal failure.
b) People with diabetes need to have good control of their blood pressure & blood sugar levels to reduce the risk of developing these problems.

Increased risk of Heart Disease & Stroke

a) Build-up of cholesterol (atherosclerosis) on the linings of the blood vessels restrict the flow of blood through the vessels which can lead to heart attack & strokes.

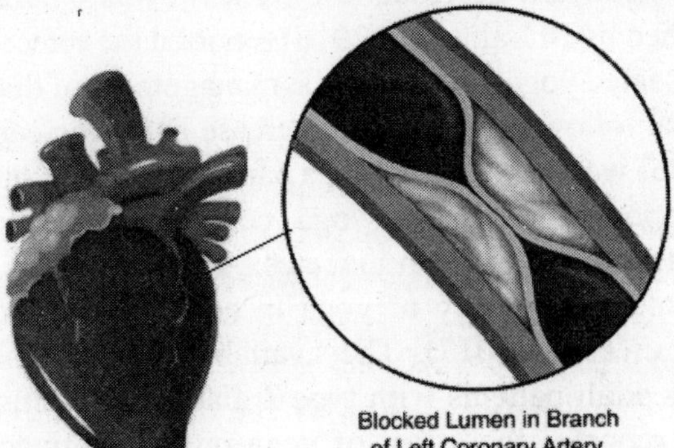

Blocked Lumen in Branch of Left Coronary Artery

Foot problems

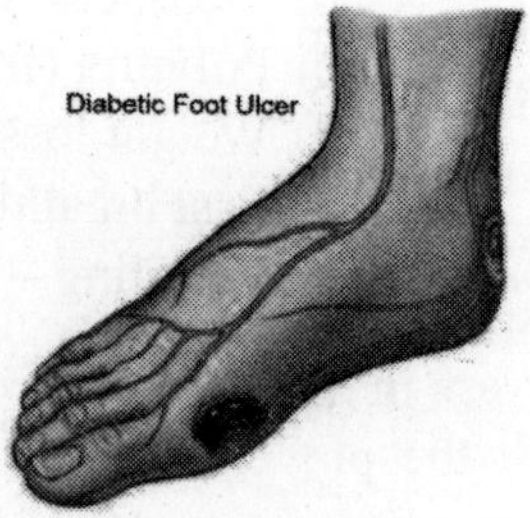

a) Diabetic Neuropathy, damage to the nerve supply to the feet which affect blood supply to the legs & feet, leading to reduced/ slow healing of any injuries.
b) Risk can be reduced by maintaining diabetic control and good foot care.

Monitoring Control of Diabetes and prevention by Yoga

a) Regular yoga session.
b) Blood glucose measurement
c) Completing blood glucose diary
d) Safe disposal of sharps

Scientific evidences for prevention of diabetes by yoga

A study published by VV et al (2017) reported the effect of short-term yoga-based lifestyle intervention on plasma glucose levels in individuals with diabetes and pre-diabetes in the community. A total of 1292 subjects with type 2 diabetes and pre-diabetes were recruited from different States of India. Yoga-based lifestyle intervention was introduced through 10-day non-residential camps. Baseline and post intervention assessments of fasting plasma glucose (FPG) were measured on the first day and tenth day respectively. The data obtained as Mean baseline FPG level was 133.1 (±47.98) and the mean post intervention FPG reduced to 121.19 (±40.56). A statistically significant decrease in FPG level was obtained. Another study published by Murali et al. (2016) reported the effect of impact of a 10 minute seated yoga practice in the management of diabetes. At a 3 month clinical follow up, the mean decrease in fasting capillary blood glucose (CBG) was 45% among yoga participants. The study provides evidence supporting the use of yoga, combined with standard care, to improve health outcomes in diabetes. A meta-analysis was carried out to evaluate the efficacy of yoga in adults with type 2 diabetes mellitusby Cui et al (2017), The available evidence suggests that yoga benefits adult patients with type 2 diabetes mellitus. Chimkode et al (2015) reported the effect of yoga on blood glucose levels in patients with type 2 diabetes mellitus. Authors reported that yoga is effective in reducing the blood glucose levels in patients with Type 2 diabetes. Beena and Sreekumaran (2013) studied the effects of yoga on curtailing the type 2 diabetes in geriatric patients. The participants in the test group showed statistically significant decrease in glucose after yogic practice. Therefore, yoga may improve risk profiles induced by stress in geriatric patients with type 2 diabetes and may have promise for the prevention or delay in diabetes complications. A significant improvement can be achieved by yogic practice in geriatric diabetes.

Yoga: for prevention of diabetes

Diabetes, a lifestyle disease, is becoming an epidemic worldwide. Along with other forms of exercise, Yoga helps a lot to control and prevent diabetes. The yogic asanas in many postures massages the pancreas and stimulates the production of insulin.

Following yoga postures will help diabetics and the people who are at high risk of diabetes:

1. Bhujangasan

This yoga posture is of a particular benefit for the diabetic patients, and is one of the primary yoga poses for the prevention and cure of diabetes.

Procedure

- Lie down on abdomen with legs close together to the ground.
- Place hands besides the body with palm touching on ground. Lift the prone body from the ground up to the naval region.

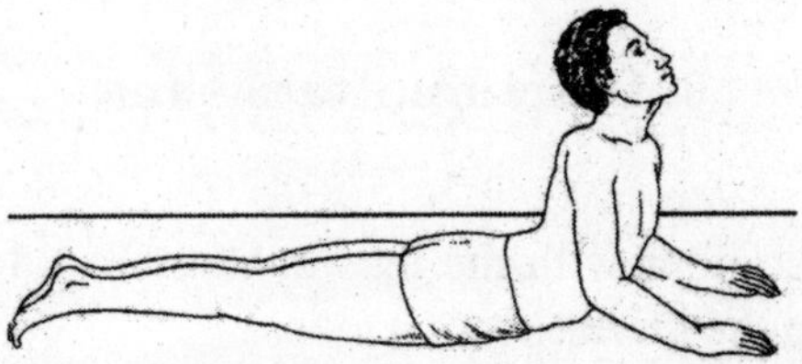

Benefits: Bhujangasana stimulates the pancreas enhancing its performance and thus, useful for people suffering from diabetes. This pose allows more blood to circulate in the body, making the organs healthy so as to perform its regular functions more effectively. Regular practice controls the blood plasma glucose level and prevents diabetes.

2. Pawanmuktasana

Procedure

It is performed first with the right lower limb, then with the left and then with both the lower limbs together. Lie on your back with your feet together and arms beside your body.

1. Lie down on your back and extend the legs and arms.
2. With exhale, draw both of your knees to your chest. Clasp your hands around your knees.
3. While holding only your right knee, release your left leg and extend it along the floor. Hold this pose for 30 seconds to 1 minute.

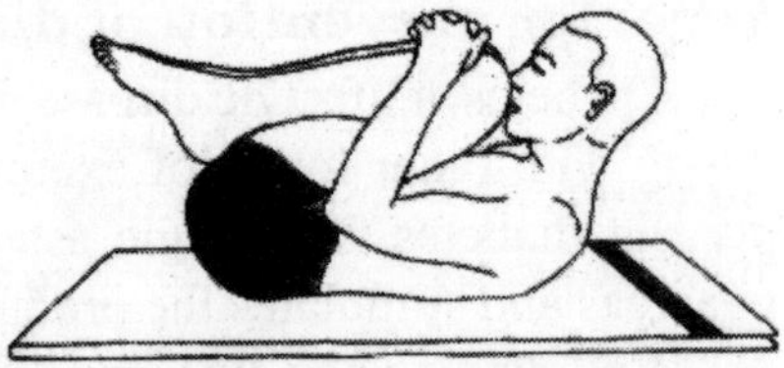

4. Draw your left knee back in towards your chest and clasp your hands around both knees again.
5. While holding only your left knee, release your right leg and extend it along the floor. Hold this pose for the same amount of time.
6. Finally, draw both knees to your chest.

Benefits: Pawanamuktasana benefits for diabetes, it helps to strengthen the liver, spleen, pancreas and abdomen along with the abdominal muscles. It is also a great exercise for strengthening and toning the back muscles. Moreover, it also helps to release flatulence from the abdomen by eliminating all the excess gas from the body.

3. Paschimottanasana

Procedure

1. Sit on the floor with the legs outstretched, feet together and hands on the knees.
2. Slowly bend forward from the hips, sliding the hands down the legs. Try to grasp the big toes with the fingers and thumbs.
3. Move slowly without forcing or jerking. Hold the position for a few seconds. Relax the back and leg muscles, allowing them to gently stretch.

4. Keeping the legs straight and utilizing the arm muscles, not the back muscles, begin to bend the elbows and gently bring the trunk down towards the legs, maintaining a firm grip on the toes, feet or legs.
5. Try to touch the knees with the forehead.

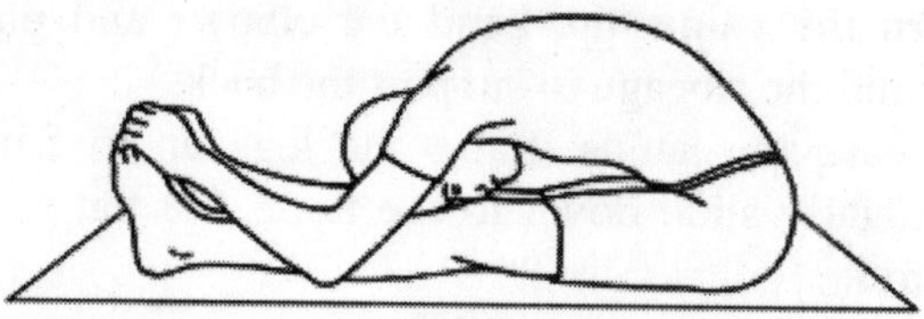

Benefits: Paschimottanasana helps prevents diabetes it helps by way of massaging the upper and lower quadrant of the abdomen including all organs such as the kidneys, adrenals, liver, pancreas, spleen and intestines.

4. Dhanurasana

Procedure

1. Lie flat on the stomach with the legs and feet together and the arms and hands beside the body.
2. Bend the knees and bring the heels close to the buttocks. Clasp the hands around the ankles. Place the chin on the floor.

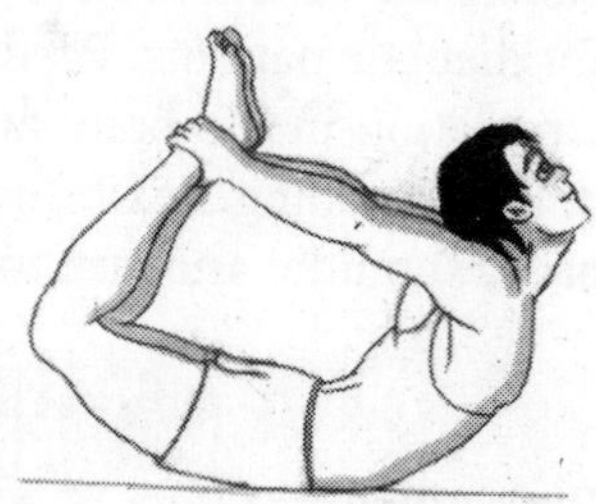

3. Tense the leg muscles and push the feet away from the body. Arch the back, lifting the thighs, chest and head together. Keep the arms straight. In the final position the head is tilted back and the abdomen supports the entire body on the floor.

Benefits: It helps to maintain a strong digestive system which directly or indirectly helps in maintaining the hormonal levels thus controlling diabetes. It also helps in reducing abdominal fat to shape body slim and improves the flexibility of spine and body posture.

5. Halasan

Procedure

- Lie flat on the back with the legs and feet together. Place the arms beside the body with the palms facing down.

- Raise both legs to the vertical position, keeping them straight and together.
- Press down on the arms and lift the buttocks, rolling the back away from the floor. Lower the legs over the head. Bring the toes towards the floor behind the head.
- Turn the palms up, bend the elbows and place the hands behind the ribcage to support the back.
- Release the hands. Raise the legs up to Sarvangasanaand gradually slide down to the floor. Lie flat on the back and relax.

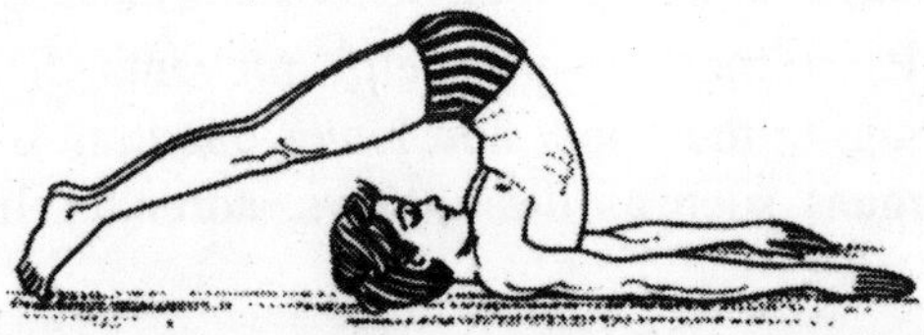

Benefits: This yoga pose is useful for maintaining a healthy pancreatic function. Arms and legs are the common areas of problems for diabetic patients. Performing Halasana helps to improve the blood circulation in the body and specifically in the arms and legs. It also helps providing flexibility to the neck and the spine, strengthen the back, shoulder and arm muscles.

6. Ardhamatsyendrasana

Procedure

1. Sit in Vajrasana position or sit straight with stretching your legs in front of you.
2. Bend your left leg and try to touch your feet to your right buttock as shown in the image.
3. Bring your right leg outside of the left knee. Touch your feet to the ground. Keep your spine erect.
4. Exhale and turn your upper body to the right. Hold your right feet with left hand and place your right hand behind you are on the ground as shown in the image.

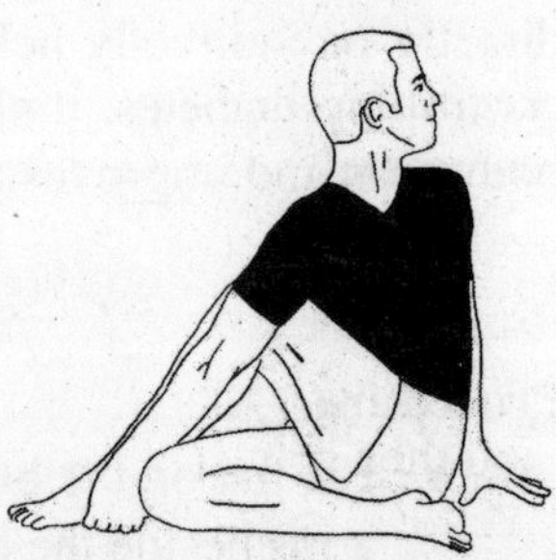

5. Breathe normally and hold this posture for 20 to 30 seconds. After practicing you can hold this posture for 3 to 5 minutes.
6. Now release this posture and repeat this cycle with bending right leg and bringing left leg outside of the right knee. (i.e. Twisting the opposite direction).

Benefits: The benefits of this asana can be felt particularly by the spinal nerves, ligaments and digestive system. Ardha Matsyendrasana gently massages the kidney and the liver and ensures improvement over backache and pain in the hips. The gentle massage in the liver ensures proper functioning and secretion of the hormones, digestion and thus the production of the insulin hormone that regulates the sugar levels in the blood.

7. Suryanamaskar

Step 1: The first step to do this pose is the Pranamasana or the Prayer Pose. This is done by:

- Standing at edge of mat and keeping the feet together, balancing the weight equally on both feet.
- Expand the chest and relax the shoulders.
- While inhaling, lift both arms upwards from sides and when exhaling bring the palms together in front of chest as when doing a prayer.

Step 2: The next step is to do the Hastauttanasana or the Raised Arms Pose

This is done when breathing air in and then lifting arms up and back, all the while keeping the biceps close to ears. The aim of this pose is to stretch the whole body up, from heels to fingertips.

Step 3: The next step is the Hasta Padasana or the Hand to Foot Pose

When exhaling, try to bend forwards from waist all the while keeping the spine straight. After finishing out the exhalation completely, bring hands down to floor besides the feet.

Step 4: The next step is to do the Ashwa Sanchalanasana or the Equestrian Pose

While inhaling air, push the left leg backwards as far as possible and then bring right knee to the floor and try to look up.

Step 5: The next step is to do Dandasana or the Stick Pose

With inhalation, take left leg backwards and bring whole body in a straight line.

Step 6: The next step is to do Ashtanga Namaskara.

To do this, gently bring the knees down to floor and breathe out. Move the hips backwards a little bit and now slide forward resting the chest and chin on floor. Raise the posterior side of your body a bit such that your both hands, both feet, both knees, chest, and chin are touching the floor.

Step 7: The next step is to do Bhujangasana or the Cobra Pose

In this, slide forward and raise your chest up into a Cobra posture. The elbows may be kept bent when doing in this pose. The shoulders need to be away from ears. Now, try and look upwards.

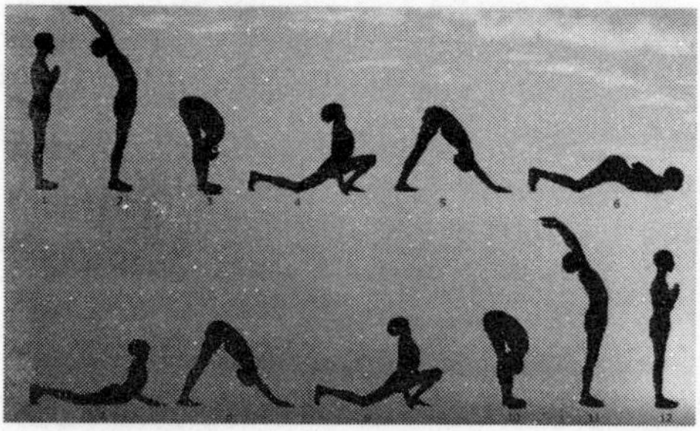

Step 8: Now, we do the Parvatasana or the Mountain Pose

Exhaling, we lift the hips and tailbone upwards and move the chest downwards in an inverted "V" shape.

Step 9: Now, we do the Hasta Padasana or the Hand to Foot Pose

Exhaling, bring left foot forward keeping palms on floor. The knees can be bent if required.

Step 10: Next step is to do Hastauttanasana or Raised Arms Pose

In this, while breathing in the spine goes up, the hands go up, and the body is bent backwards slightly, pushing hips a little bit in the outward direction.

Step 11: The last step is to do the Tadasana

In this, while exhaling, the body needs to be straightened first and the arms should be brought down. Now, relax in this position and try and observe sensations passing through your body.

Step 12: Pranamasan

Benefits: Surya Namaskar is a helpful Yogasanaas it helps in stimulation of insulin in our body. Surya Namaskar also helps in increasing the blood supply to various parts of our body and provides benefits if practiced at 4 rounds per minute.

Pranayam

Kapalbhati: The individuals having high diabetes should practice for 10-30 minutes daily in the morning and evening on an empty stomach.

Procedure

1. Sit in Padmasana, put both hands on respective knees. Exhale faster and forcibly through both the nostrils. Simultaneously draw the abdomen in.
2. After completing exhalation with force, take the breath in and bring the abdomen in previous position.
3. The sound produced during inhalation and exhalation should be like a bellows of the blacksmith.

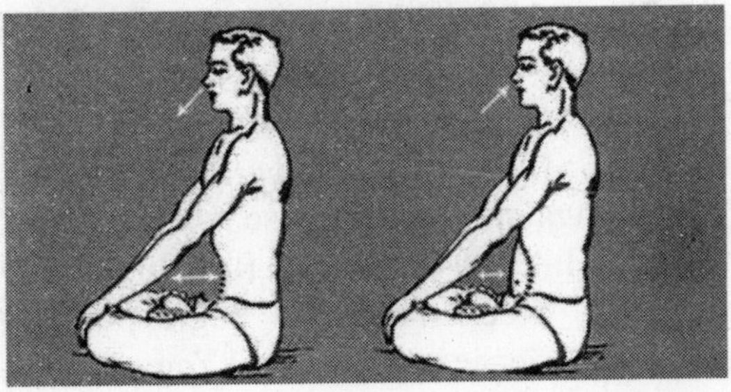

Benefits: Daily practice of Kapalbhati improves the function and strength of the pancreas. It regenerates the beta cells of the pancreas. Regular practice cures diabetes also. This Pranayam is very effective in lowering the blood glucose.

Anulom-Viloma (Alternate Nostril Breathing)

Procedure

1. Sit in Padmasana with head and spine erect and eyes closed.
2. Close the right nostrils with the right thumb.

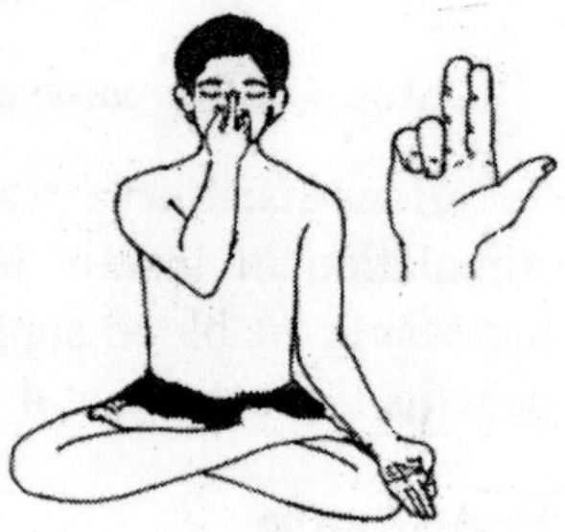

3. Inhale through the left nostril just before closing it with ring finger and release the air through the right nostril.
4. Repeat the process alternatively for both the nostrils about 5 times without making any sound.

Benefits: Calms and steadies the mind. Improves focus and concentration. Manages hypertension. Helps to prevent diabetes and keeps diabetes under control.

References

1. V V, Rathi A, Raghuram N. Effect of short-term yoga-based lifestyle intervention on plasma glucose levels in individuals with diabetes and pre-diabetes in the community. Diabetes Metab Syndr. 2017 Apr 12. pii: S1871-4021(17)30083-8.
2. Mullur RS, Ames D. Impact of a 10 minute Seated Yoga Practice in the Management of Diabetes. J Yoga Phys Ther. 2016 Jan 18; 6(1).
3. Cui J, Yan JH, Yan LM, Pan L, Le JJ, Guo YZ. Effects of yoga in adults with type 2 diabetes mellitus: A meta-analysis. J Diabetes Investing. 2017 Mar; 8(2):201-209.
4. Chimkode SM, Kumaran SD, Kanhere VV, Shivanna R. Effect of yoga on blood glucose levels in patients with type 2 diabetes mellitus. J Clin Diagn Res. 2015 Apr; 9 (4): CC01-3.
5. Beena RK, Sreekumaran E. Yogic practice and diabetes mellitus in geriatric patients. Int J Yoga. 2013 Jan; 6(1):47-54.

❐

16
Yoga for Prevention of Osteoporosis

As per the definition of osteoporosis by World Health Organization, osteoporosis is a generalized skeletal disorder of low bone mass (thinning of the bone) and deterioration in its architecture, causing susceptibility to fracture. Osteoporosis occurs because the rate of bone formation is lower than bone resorption.

Bone consists of a thick outer shell and a strong inner mesh filled with collagen (protein), calcium salts and other minerals. The inside looks like honeycomb, with blood vessels and bone marrow in the spaces between bones.

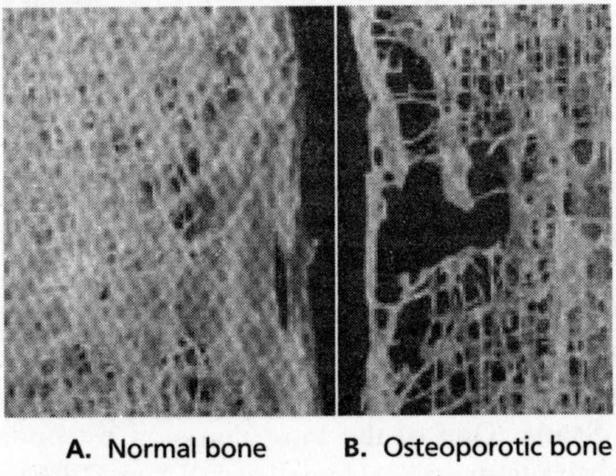

A. Normal bone B. Osteoporotic bone

Epidemiology

Osteoporosis is worldwide prevalent and serious public health concern. A report from International osteoporosis foundation suggests that over 200 million people worldwide suffer with this disease.

The incidence of osteoporosis will be rapidly increasing due to increased life expectancy and hence ageing. The incidence is higher in the women of post-menopausal age. India with 1.25 billion people and the second most populated country in the world have approximately 10% of population aged above 50 years. A recent study reports that approximately 50 million people in India are either osteoporotic (T-score lower than – 2.5) or have low bone mass (T-score between – 1.0 and – 2.5) (Mithal and Kaur, 2012).

Primary cause of osteoporosis

Osteoporosis results from an imbalance between two normal activities of bone: bone resorption and bone formation. There are two types of cells in bone 1. Osteoblast, which is responsible for bone formation and 2. Osteoclast, which is responsible for bone resorption i.e. the process by which osteoclasts break down the tissue in bones and release the minerals, resulting in a transfer of calcium from bone tissue to the blood. The combined processes of bone resorption and bone formation allow the healthy skeleton to be maintained continually by the removal of old bone and its replacement with new bone. These combined processes are referred to as bone remodeling or bone turnover. During the first 20-25 years of life, these processes are balanced. When the destruction of bone begins to exceed the formation of bone to a net loss of bone begins. The risk of fracture increases from 1.5 to 3-fold for every 10% decrease in bone mass.

Diagnosis of osteoporosis

Bone mineral density test: A bone mineral density test, detects osteoporosis. It estimates how dense or thick your bones are by using X-rays. The X-rays measure how much calcium and minerals are in a part of your bone. The more minerals you have, the better would be your bones. The lower your mineral content, the greater risk of osteoporosis.

DEXA Scans: One of the most common osteoporosis tests is dual X-ray absorptiometry - also called DXA or DEXA. It measures people's spine, hip, or total-body bone density to help gauge their risk of fractures.

Bone density which is 2.5 SD or more below the young normal mean (T score < – 2.5) may be classified as showing osteoporosis, while a BMD T score between –1 and –2.5 may be classified as showing osteopenia.

Risk factors for osteoporosis

The risk factors which may contribute to osteoporosis are:

a. **Age:** The bone density reaches maximum level around age 30. Thereafter, the person lose bone mass. Therefore one should more cautious for strengthening the bones by taking proper diet and exercise.
b. **Gender:** Men and women are both at risk of osteoporosis however women are more likely to have the osteoporosis.
c. **Family history:** Persons with family history of fractured hip may likely to have osteoporosis.
d. **Ethnicity:** Caucasian and Asian women are more likely to have osteoporosis than women of other ethnic backgrounds. There bone mass and density compared with other ethnic groups are lower hence they are more prone to osteoporosis.
e. **Diseases like rheumatoid arthritis:** Rheumatoid arthritis may increase the rate of osteoporosis.
f. **Smoking and alcohol:** Smoking and alcohol may lead to thinning of bones and therefore make the person more prone to osteoporosis.

Vegetarian foods that prevent osteoporosis

Vegeterian diet rich in calcium and Vitamin D can be helpful in preventing osteoporosis. Examples are brocolli, cabbage, cauliflower, beetroot, okra (ladies' finger), ragi, dates have calcium and magnesium. Fruits with vitamin C: oranges, guava, strawberries, and pineapples, mustard green, turnip greens and pulses.

Yoga prevents osteoporosis: scientific evidences

Fishman (2009) performed a study on eighteen women patients with osteoporosis or osteopenia with average age 68 years. Yoga was performed daily for 10 minutes for two years. Pre and post yoga DEXA scan was performed. Results showed that yoga practitioners gained 0.76 and 0.94 points for spine and hips, respectively, on the T-scale when compared with controls. The author has concluded that yoga appears to be an effective way to build bone mineral density after menopause. After the pilot study was successful, Dr. Fishman made a DVD and gave it away to 1000 people from every part of the world to use for their next study. It took eight years to get all the data to complete his second study. Dr. Fishman published this 1000 patient study in Geriatric and rehabilitation journal that twelve-minute daily yoga regimen reverses osteoporotic bone loss (Lu et al. (2016)).

Improvement in BMD could be attributed to the effects of mechano-transduction which plays an important role in pathologic fracture healing, physical adaptations, and most importantly the therapeutic adaptations to osteogenesis (Huang and Ogawa, 2010). In order to meet the functional demands in the mechanical environment, physical remodeling of the bone takes place. There is a dynamic balance maintained between the process osteogenesis and bone resorption by the virtue of mechanical loading which activates the mechano-transducers to do so (Huang and Ogawa, 2010). Effects of Yogasanas on osteoporosis in postmenopausal women were published by Motorwala et al. (They reported the improvement in T-score of DEXA scan of -2.55 ± 0.25 at post-training as compared to a pre-training score of -2.69 ± 0.17). The study concluded that integrated yoga is a safe mode of physical activity which includes weight bearing as well as not weight bearing asanas, Pranayama, and SuryaNamaskar, all of which helps induce improvement in BMD in postmenopausal osteoporotic females. Sparrowe (2001) reported that yoga has ability to stimulate the bones to retain calcium, provided the body gets enough calcium in the first place. The retaining of calcium occurs through weight bearing poses of Yogasana. Phoosuwan et. al (2009) published their study in the Journal of Medical Association of Thailand and reported that weight bearing yoga training has shown a positive effect on the bone by reducing the bone resorption and hence preventing the risk of osteoporosis in postmenopausal women. Grabara and Szopa (2010) studied effects of Yogasanas on spine flexibility in women over 50 years old. Authors concluded that Yogasanas make muscles more flexible and to increase the range of motion in the joints, which is particularly important for improving their life quality. It has positive effects on patients ailing with back pain, arthritis, and issues related to increased risk of falls, which might lead to osteoporotic fractures (Sherman *et al.,* 2005). It helps improve the overall quality of life of an individual.

The scientific evidences suggest that yoga improves in BMD and integrated yoga exercises should be an important component of any osteoporosis treatment exercise regime.

Yoga regimen for prevention of osteoporosis

The yoga regimen described here are extremely beneficial in prevention of osteoporosis and osteopenia. The elderly may practice these yoga regimens to strengthen their bones. The procedure of these yoga postures and benefits are given below:

1. Vrikshasana (Tree pose)

Procedure: Stand erects on the left leg, bend the right leg and place the right foot on the root of right thigh. Maintain the pose like as a tree on the ground. This is called vriksha-asana.

Benefits: It improves balancing skill on one foot, strengthens the muscles of the lower limbs.

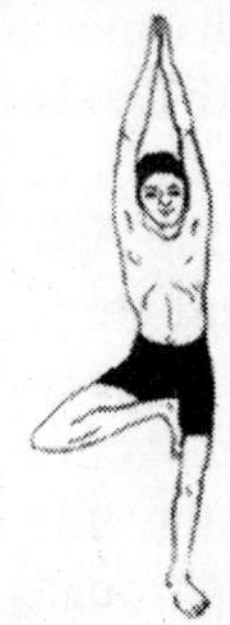

2. Trikonasana

Procedure

1. Stand erect and keep distance between your legs about 3 to 4 feet.
2. Extend your arms at the shoulder level.
3. Inhale and raises your right arm by the side of your head.
4. Now, bend your right arms with exhaling towards the left side by keeping your body weight equally on both the feet. You should ensure that the right arm become parallel to the ground.

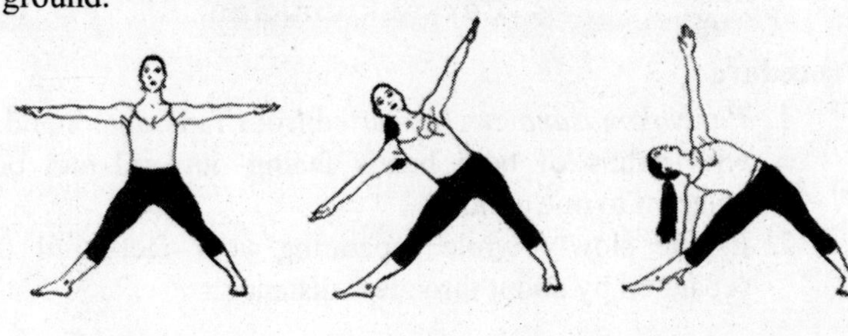

5. Maintain the position as per your comfort with normal breathing (for 5-10 seconds) and come back to the original position by inhaling.
6. Do the same procedure with the left arm.

Benefits: This asana tones up the muscles in trunk, legs and hips, improves the flexibility of spine, relieves the pain in the neck and back.

3. Virbhadrasana type II

Procedure

First get into the standing position keep your body straight. Keep a distance of 3-4 feet between each foot. Breathe in and lift up your both hands. (Keep your hands parallel to the floor or ground) and turn your head to the right side. During breathing out gently turn your right feet at the angle of 90 degrees to the right side. Now gently bend your right knee little bit downward to the ground. Ensure that your right thigh ought to be parallel to the floor. Remain in this Pose for 30 seconds and breathe deeply about 3 to 4 times. After that breathe out and slowly down your hands and come to the standing position and breathe normally. Rest for a while.

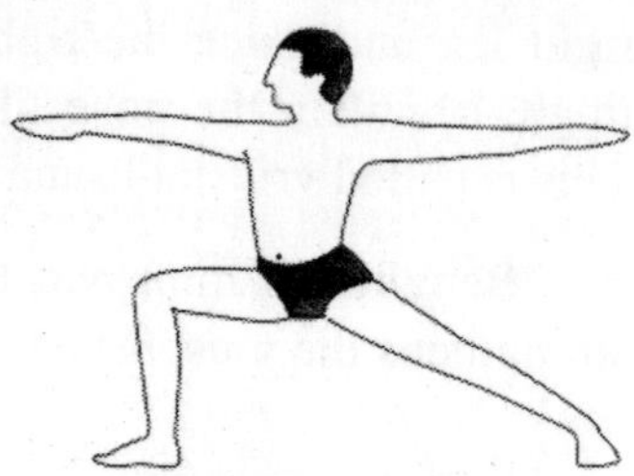

After this attempt the same steps with your left leg by turning your head to the left side. Repeat this process for 3 to 6 times.

Benefits: This Pose stretches and strengthens legs and ankles. It helps to stretch the chest, lungs and shoulders. It helps to boost the stamina. Relieves in any kind of backaches. It is beneficial in the problems of osteoporosis, flat feet, carpal tunnel syndrome and infertility.

4. Parsvakonasana

Procedure

1. *Parsvakonasana* can be started from Tadasana. Stand straight with palms of both hands facing outward and both feel adjacent to one another.
2. Exhale slowly while separating your feet until they are separated by about three feet distance.

3. Now raise your hands so that they are at the sides fully stretched and parallel to the floor. In this position, your shoulders should remain wide, the feet should be kept apart and the palms facing down.
4. Turn your left foot towards the left side, while the right foot still faces forward.
5. Turn the left thigh inwards until the ankle and the center of the left knee of your left foot are in a straight line.
6. Turn the hip slightly towards your left leg but your chest should remain straight.
7. Bend the left knee over your left ankle while inhaling, so that your shin is perpendicular to the floor.
8. The left thigh should also remain parallel to the ground with the right leg remaining straight and stretched fully from hip to ankle.
9. Now extend and stretch the right hand above your head on the left side of your body, with the palm facing the ground and remaining straight. The hand should be touching your right ear.

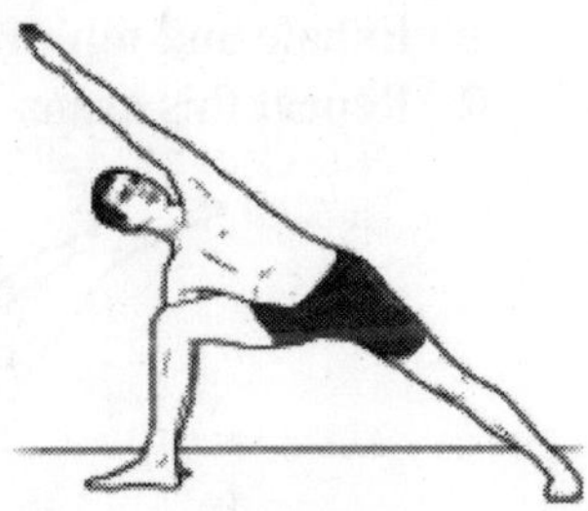

10. Turn your face slowly inward to look at your palm. The other hand should be touching the ankle of your left leg without taking any support from the ankle or the shoulder. The purpose of Parsvakonasana is to stretch as much towards the right side of your body as possible without feeling any discomfort.
11. Push your extended hand towards the ceiling forcefully, while inhaling and exhaling. Repeat this stretching a few times and then return back to standing position.
12. Repeat the same steps with the right leg.

Benefits: It provides stretching of many body parts, helping the legs, chest, lungs, ankles, spine, shoulders and abdomen. This pose strengthens the knees, ankles and legs while stretching muscles in the, abdomen, lungs, chest and waist. It increases stamina. It is beneficial in prevention of osteoporosis.

5. Shalabhasana

Procedure

1. Lie down on the floor on your belly and place your chin on the floor.
2. Place your toes on the floor; touch the knees to the ground.
3. Place your hands below the hips on the ground below your hips in a way that your palms rest on the ground.
4. While inhaling lift up your head, upper body, thighs and legs off the floor.
5. Raise your leg as high as possible, hold your breath and remain in this position resting your body on your belly.
6. Exhale and return to the starting position.
7. Repeat this asana 10 times.

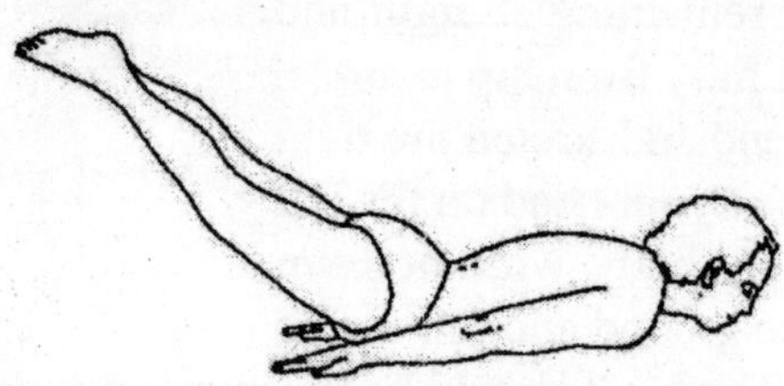

Benefits: This pose develops self-confidence and invigorates the body as the internal organs are stimulated and the acid-base balance of your body is regulated. Performing this asana strengthens your leg, pelvic arms, shoulders, thighs, calf muscles and hips and back muscles. The locust pose encourages good posture and a slim figure. It is beneficial for prevention of osteoporosis and osteopenia.

6. Setubandhasana

Procedure

1. Begin the asana by lying flat on your back.
2. Bend your knees and place your feet on the floor hip-width apart. Make sure that your ankles and knees are placed in a straight line.
3. Let your arms rest beside your body, with your palms facing downwards.
4. Inhale, and lift your back (lower, upper, and middle) off the floor. Roll in your shoulders, and make sure your chin touches

your chest without you having to move it. Let your shoulders, feet, and arms support your weight.

5. Firm up your buttocks as you tighten them. Make sure your thighs are parallel to each other and the floor.
6. Interlace your fingers and push your hands harder to the ground to lift your torso higher.
7. Hold the posture for at least a minute. Breathe slowly and deeply.
8. Exhale and release the pose.

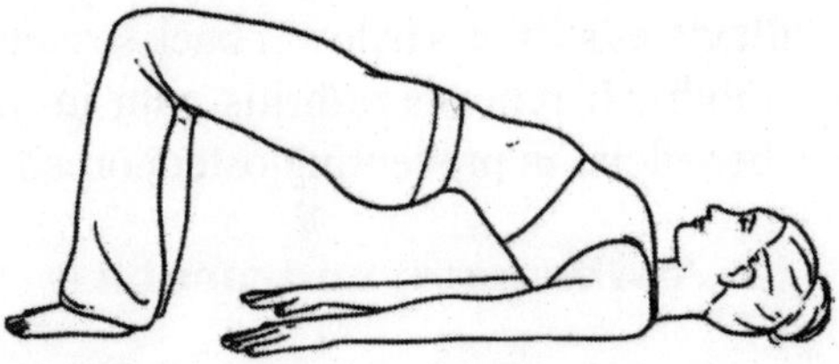

Benefits: This asana helps to strengthen the muscles of the back. The stretch also helps to relieve the stress trapped in the back. This asana stretches and tones the neck, spine, and chest. With regular practice of this asana, blood circulation is also improved. It is beneficial in preventing osteoporosis and osteopenia.

7. Suptapadangusthasana

Procedure

1. Lie down on your back with your legs stretched out and feet flexed. Press your feet through your heels.
2. By exhaling pull your right knee towards your chest, and loop a strap around the arch of the right foot. If you are a seasoned yoga practitioner, use two fingers and hook them onto the big toe.
3. Straighten and stretch your right leg up to the ceiling, such that your arms are straight, and your shoulders are pressing the floor.
4. Keep pushing and extending your left leg, pressing the top of your left thigh down with the left hand. The extension of the right leg must create a comfortable stretch in the back of the leg.

5. You could either hold the pose here or turn the right leg out, bringing that leg down on your right side. But if you do this, you must ensure your left hip is grounded on the floor.

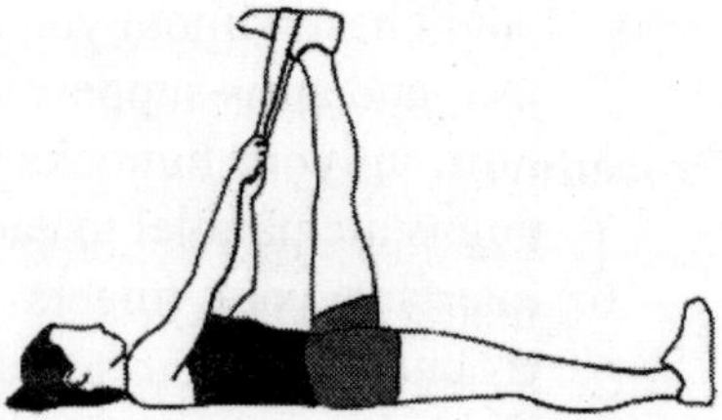

6. Hold each variation for as long as you are comfortable, and then repeat the asana with the left leg on top.

Benefits: It alleviates stiffness in lower back stretches hamstrings, calves, and inner thighs. It relieves arthritis pain in hips and knees, aligns pelvis. It is beneficial in preventing osteoporosis.

8. Ardhamatsyendrasana

Procedure

1. Sit in Vajrasana position or sit straight with stretching your legs in front of you.
2. Bend your left leg and try to touch your feet to your right buttock as shown in the image.
3. Bring your right leg outside of the left knee. Touch your feet to the ground. Keep your spine erect.
4. Exhale and turn your upper body to the right. Hold your right feet with left hand and place your right hand behind you are on the ground as shown in the image.
5. Breathe normally and hold this posture for 20 to 30 seconds. After practicing you can hold this posture for 3 to 5 minutes.

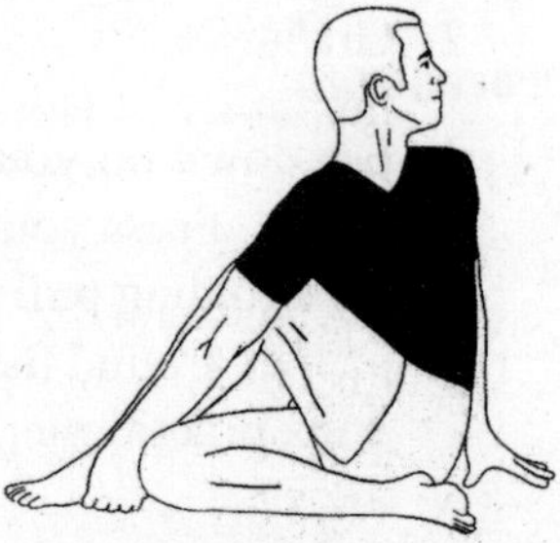

6. Now release this posture and repeat this cycle with bending right leg and bringing left leg outside of the right knee. (i.e. Twisting the opposite direction).

Benefits: It strengthens the spinal column and muscles of the back. This asana is beneficial in preventing osteoporosis and osteopenia.

9. Shavasana

Procedure

1. Lie down on back and place hands near the thighs and palm facing upwards.
2. Keep the heels slightly apart and toes pointing outwards with relaxed body.
3. Maintain the position for 5-10 seconds or as long as comfortable.

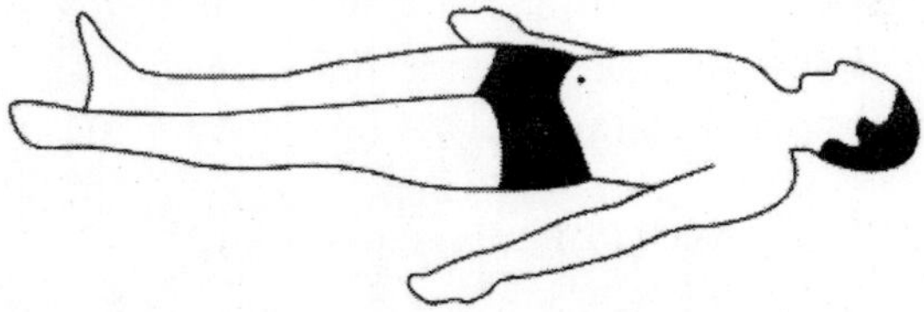

Benefits: Relaxes whole body. Relieves physical and mental fatigue. Extremely beneficial for relieving stress. Beneficial in preventing osteoporosis.

References

1. Fishman, L. Yoga for Osteoporosis: A Pilot Study. Topics in Geriatric Rehabilitation: 2009; 25: 244–250.
2. Grabara M, Szopa J. Effects of hatha yoga exercises on spine flexibility in women over 50 years old. J Phys Ther Sci. 2015 Feb; 27(2):361-5.
3. Huang C, Ogawa R. Mechanotransduction in bone repair and regeneration. FASEB J. 2010 Oct; 24(10):3625-32.
4. Lu, Yi-Hsueh; Rosner, B; Chang, G; Fishman, L. Twelve-minute daily yoga regimen reverses osteoporotic bone loss. Topics in Geriatric Rehabilitation: April/June 2016; 32: 81–87.
5. Mithal A, Kaur P. Osteoporosis in Asia: A call to action. Curr Osteoporos Rep. 2012;10:245–7.
6. Motorwala ZS, Kolke S, Panchal PY, Bedekar NS, Sancheti PK, Shyam A. Effects of Yogasanas on osteoporosis in postmenopausal women. Int J Yoga. 2016 Jan-Jun; 9(1):44-8.
7. Phoosuwan M, Kritpet T, Yuktanandana P. The effects of weight bearing yoga training on the bone resorption markers

of the postmenopausal women. J Med Assoc Thai. 2009 Sep; 92 Suppl5:S102-8.
8. Sherman KJ, Cherkin DC, Erro J, Miglioretti DL, Deyo RA. Comparing yoga,exercise, and a self-care book for chronic low back pain: a randomized,controlled trial. Ann Intern Med. 2005 Dec 20;143(12):849-56.
9. Sparrowe L. Good to the bone. Yoga J. 2001. p. 112.

❐

17

Yoga as a Preventive Therapy for Rheumatoid Arthritis

Yoga: Yoga is a system of lifestyle, philosophy and practices, which helps evolve the person's potentials, including the physical, vital, mental, emotional, psychic and spiritual qualities. Yoga covers a broad range of techniques applicable to all aspects of life. The attainment of sensory control through self-restraint and self-realization through meditation has become the aspiration for a large number of people, propelled to some extent by the belief that the human body and human mind have the ability to prevent and cure disease and achieve a state of well-being given the right tools e. g. yoga. This article emphasizes the effects of yoga on human inflammatory diseases in particular rheumatoid arthritis.

Effect of Yoga on Inflammation

Inflammation is a protective immune response mounted by the innate immune system in response to harmful stimuli, such as pathogens, tissue damage, dead cells or irritants, and is tightly regulated by the host immune system. Tissue damage causes release of vasoactive and chemotactic factors that trigger a local increase in blood flow and capillary permeability. Permeable capillaries allow an influx of fluid and cells. Phagocytic cells migrate to the site of inflammation by the process known as chemotaxis and phagocytes and antibacterial exudates destroy the bacteria.

Inflammation can be classified as i) acute inflammation, which occurs over seconds, minutes, hours, and days, ii) chronic inflammation, which occurs over longer period of time. Acute inflammation is a healthy physiological response indicative of wound healing while chronic inflammation has been directly implicated in a wide range of human health disorders encompassing almost all present day diseases including auto-immune diseases, obesity, diabetes and atherosclerosis, similar to the onset of inflammation, the resolution of inflammation is an intricate and active process. Can we therefore harness the mediators involved in resolution responses by yoga to treat patients with chronic inflammatory or autoimmune diseases?

Differences between acute and chronic inflammation

Features	Acute inflammation	Chronic inflammation
Onset	Fast: minutes or hours	Slow: days
Cellular infiltrates	Neutrophils	Monocytes/acrophages/ lymphocytes
Fibrosis/Tissue injury	Usually mild and self limited	Often severe and progressive
Local and systemic signs	Prominent	Less prominent; may be subtle

The literatures published suggest that yoga can diminish the inflammation in variety of chronic inflammatory diseases.

Yoga is Beneficial in Rheumatoid Arthritis (RA)

Rheumatoid Arthritis (RA) is an autoimmune disease in which the body's own immune system mistakenly attacks the joints. This creates inflammation that causes the tissue that lines the inside of joints (the synovium) to thicken, resulting in swelling and pain in and around the joints. The synovium makes a fluid that lubricates joints and helps them move smoothly. If inflammation goes unchecked, it can damage cartilage, the elastic tissue that covers the ends of bones in a joint, as well as the bones themselves. Over time, there is loss of cartilage, and the joint spacing between bones can become smaller. Joints can become loose, unstable, painful and lose their mobility. Joint deformity also can occur. Joint damage cannot be reversed, and because it can occur early, doctors recommend early diagnosis and aggressive treatment to control RA which may cause side effects.

Regular practice of yoga makes a big difference when you have RA. It's important to keep muscles strong to support the joints, and movement is important to reduce stiffness. Yoga can be a fun alternative to walking, swimming, biking, and other activities. Being fit also makes less likely to get heart disease and diabetes, two conditions that are more common if you have rheumatoid arthritis. A program of yoga poses, breathing, and relaxation can make a big difference in joint tenderness and swelling, according to the Arthritis Foundation.

The published reports suggests that Yoga is one of the strategy to treat RA, Badsha and Chhabra conducted an 8-week pilot study to evaluate an intervention of structured bi-weekly specially structured yoga program for rheumatoid arthritis. They looked at the impact of this program on disease activity indices, disability, quality of life, and impact on treatment. Significant benefits in disease activity scores, ability to reduce medications and, fatigue were noted (Badsha and Chhabra, 2009). Evans et al (2013) performed a study to assess the impact of a 6-week twice/week Iyengar yoga program on health-related quality of life of young adults with RA compared with a usual-care wait list control group. The study suggested that a brief Iyengar yoga intervention is a feasible and safe adjunctive treatment for young people with RA, leading to improvements in health-related quality of life, pain disability, fatigue, and mood benefits. Moreover, improvements in quality of life, pain disability, and mood persisted at the 2-month follow-up. Telles et al. (2011) reported that one week yoga practice reduced the rheumatoid factor levels and thus beneficial in RA.

Moonaz et al. (2015) reported in a clinical trial that yoga may help sedentary individuals with arthritis improve physical and psychological health and health-related quality of life (HRQOL). In this trial the objective was to evaluate the effect of Integral-based hatha yoga in sedentary people with arthritis. Total 75 sedentary adults above 18 years of age with RA or knee osteoarthritis randomly assigned to 8 weeks of yoga (two 60-min classes and 1 home practice/week) or wait list. Poses were modified for individual needs. In everyone completing yoga, we explored long-term effects at 9 months. Participants were mostly female (96%), white (55%), and college-educated (51%), with a mean (SD) age of 52 years (12 yrs). Average disease duration was 9 years and 49% had RA. At 8 weeks, yoga was associated with significantly higher physical component summary, walking capacity, and lower Center for Epidemiologic Studies Depression Scale. Significant improvements were reported in physical, pain, general health, vitality, and mental health scales. Among all yoga participants, significant improvements were observed in mean physical component summary, flexibility, 6-min walk, and all psychological and most HRQOL domains at 8 weeks with most still evident 9 months later (Moonaz *et al.,* 2015). Ranjna et al. (2015) reported that RA patients who were given naturopathy (message and hydrotherapy) along with yoga therapy resulted in decrease of RA factors and pro-inflammatory marker IL6 (Ranjna *et al.,* 2015). The Ph.D dissertation submitted by Vijay Kumar Singh (2008) found that 40 days yoga package practice lead to decreased pain in RA patients.

Table 1. Scientific evidence of effects of yoga on RA

S. No.	Yoga duration	Subject no. (n)	RA disease status	References
1.	8-week		Signicant benefits in disease activity scores, ability to reduce medications and, fatigue were noted	Badsha and Chhabra, 2009
2.	6-week	n = 26	A brief Iyengar yoga intervention is a feasible and safe adjunctive treatment for young people with RA, leading to improvements in health-related quality of life, pain disability, fatigue, and mood benefits.	Evans *et al.,* 2013
3.	One week	n = 40	Rheumatoid factor level decreased	Telles *et al.,* 2011

4.	8 weeks	n = 75	Significant improvements were observed in mean physical component summary, flexibility, 6-min walk, and all psychological and most HRQOL domains at 8 weeks with most still evident 9 months later	Moonaz *et al.*, 2015
5.	12 months	n = 39	decrease of RA factors and pro-inflammatory marker IL6	Ranjna *et al.*, 2015
6.	40 days	n = 160	decrease of CRP and pain	Singh , 2008

Yoga package described by various literatures (Ranjana et al, 2015; Singh, 2008) which is helpful in RA disease is given below:

Asanas of Anti rheumatic Series

Pawanmuktasan: It relieves pain and strengthens musculoskeletal system. It is performed first with the right lower limb, then with the left and then with both the lower limbs together. Lie on your back with your feet together and arms beside your body.

1. Lie down on your back and extend the legs and arms.
2. With exhale, draw both of your knees to your chest. Clasp your hands around your knees.
3. While holding only your right knee, release your left leg and extend it along the floor. Hold this pose for 30 seconds to 1 minute.
4. Draw your left knee back in towards your chest and clasp your hands around both knees again.

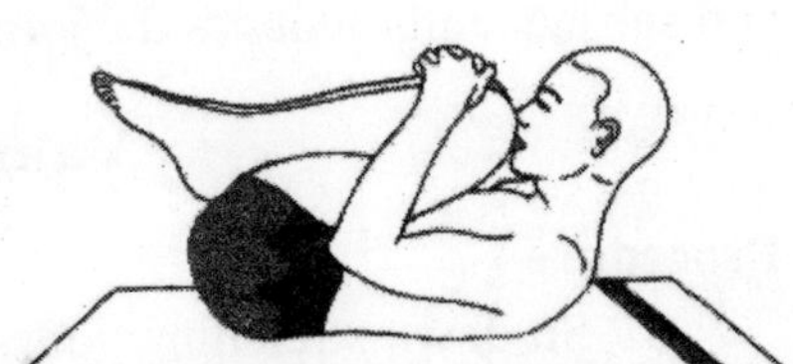

5. While holding only your left knee, release your right leg and extend it along the floor. Hold this pose for the same amount of time.
6. Finally, draw both knees to your chest.

Benefits: Performing yoga particularly Pawanmuktasana is beneficial to musculoskeletal system and helps to reduce pain, disability and improves the quality of life of the patients. Studies have also reported that patient who performs pawanmuktasana shows lower levels of pro inflammatory cytokines.

Marjari Asana

Procedure

1. Start on hands and knees with shoulders stacked over the wrists and knees directly below the hips.
2. Moving with the inhalation start to arch the back, lifting the chin and hips.
3. On the exhale press the palms into the mat, round the spine and tuck the chin to the chest.
4. Continue with this movement 3-4 times.

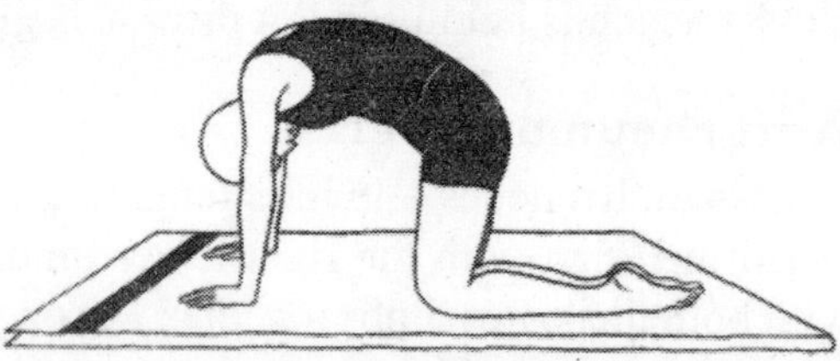

Benefits: Murjari asana is beneficial to musculoskeletal system and helps to reduce pain, and improves the quality of life of the patients. Long term practice of Murjari asana reduces the typical rheumatic symptoms. Practicing asana with mindfulness on posture and movement at joint position creates suppleness at joints, relaxes stiff muscles. Thus increasing the joint flexibility and gives mobility and subsequently reduces the joint inflammatory symptoms.

Vakrasana

Procedure

1. Sit down stretching your legs forward on the ground.
2. Keep your hands beside your thighs or buttocks.
3. Bend your right leg straight and stretched.
4. Keep the left foot beside the right knee and the left knee raised upward.

5. Inhale and raise the arms shoulder high, keeping the elbows straight.
6. Exhaling, twist to the left, place the right arm by the outer side of the left knee and hold the left ankle with the right hand.
7. Take the left hand behind the back keeping the palms on the floor.
8. Look backward towards the left side.
9. Hold on the position.
10. The final position of each stage should be held while breathing, naturally. Hold the position as long as comfortable.
11. Then inhale and raise the right arm shoulder high, keeping the elbows straight.
12. Exhaling, release the left twist, place the right hand by the side of right buttock and left hand by the side of left buttock.
13. Take a deep breath and relax.
14. Repeat the same from the other side.
15. Practice on both sides.

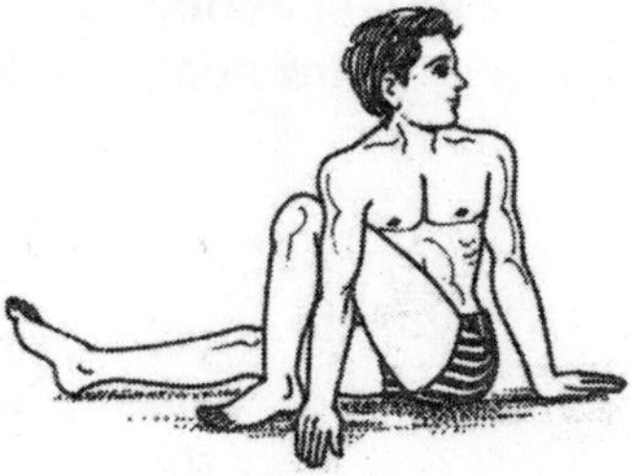

Benefits: It improves flexibility of spine, shoulders and eases back pain. Relieve the pain in arthritis.

Shashakasana

Procedure

- Sit in Vajrasana with palms on the knees.
- Raise your arms up. Stretch upwards from the trunk.
- Then keeping the arms straight, lower your body towards the floor. Rest your hands on the floor. Then try to touch either the forehead or the crown of the head on the floor. Ensure that your elbows are straight.
- Close your eyes and maintain the pose for three to five breaths.
- To come out of the asana, first lift your head off the floor, then raise the body and hands up. Slowly bring the hands down and rest them on the knees, come out of Vajrasana and sit in a relaxed manner.

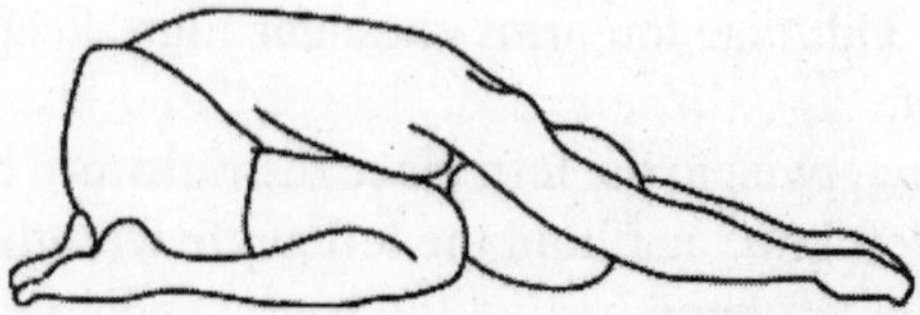

Benefits: It strengthens abdomen and stretches human back, shoulder and arm. This yogasana is beneficial to musculoskeletal system and helps to reduce pain.

Bhujangasana: In this asana, from a prone position with palms and legs on the floor, the chest is lifted.

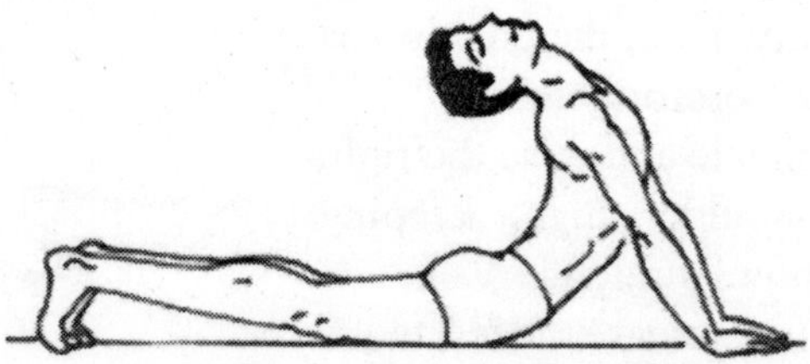

Benefits: It strengthens vertebral column and stretches theabdomen, shoulder, thorax andlLung. It is beneficial in Rheumatoid arthritis and relieves pain in joints.

Shalabhasana: It is a back bend, or spine stretch, utilizing the strength of the upper and middle back to lift the weight of the legs as high as possible from a starting position while face down on the floor.

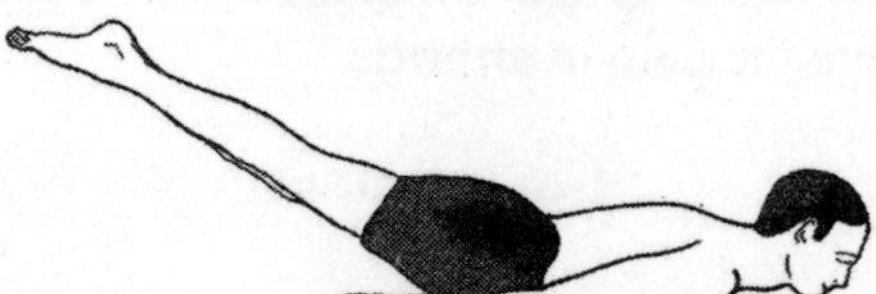

Benefits: This posture of yogasana strengthens leg, vertebral column and arms. It stretches shoulder, thorax, thigh and navel. It improves flexibility and coordination. It is beneficial in managing rheumatoid arthritis.

Halasana: The practitioner lies on the floor, lifts the legs, and then places them behind the head.

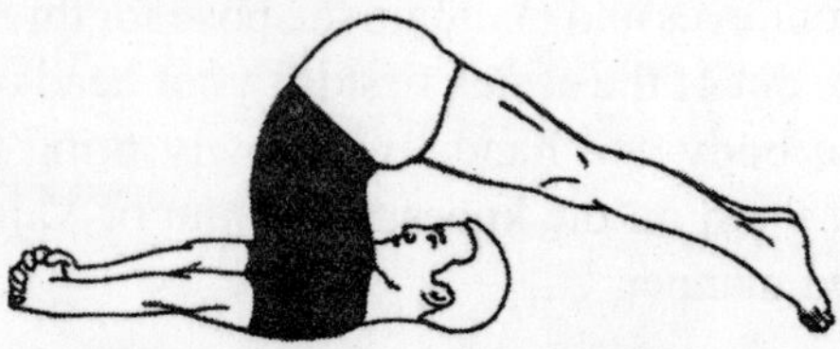

Benefits: This posture of yogasana stretches shoulder and vertebral column. It is beneficial in Rheumatoid arthritis. It relieves pain in joints and regular practice reduces inflammation in joints.

The above asana should be practiced for 40 minutes followed by Shavasana for 10 min.

Pranayamas

Anulom Vilom: 10 min- 3 round
Bhastrika pranayam: 5 min -2 round
Bhramary: 5 min -10 round

Followed by Om chanting for 10 min

In summary, over time, as the age increases there is loss of cartilage, and the joint spacing between bones can become smaller. Joints can become loose, unstable, and painful and lose their mobility. Joint deformity also can occur. Joint damage cannot be reversed, and because it can occur early. Practicing yoga regularly prevents rheumatoid as well as osteoarthritis. Consider the yogic regimen as important part of lifestyle and disease management.

References

1. Badsha H, Chhabra V, Leibman C, Mofti A, Kong KO. The benefits of yoga for rheumatoid arthritis: results of a preliminary, structured 8-week program. Rheumatol Int. 2009 Oct;29(12):1417-21.
2. Evans S, Moieni M, Lung K, Tsao J, Sternlieb B, Taylor M, Zeltzer L. Impact of iyengar yoga on quality of life in young women with rheumatoid arthritis. Clin J Pain. 2013 Nov;29 (11): 988-97.
3. Bower JE, Greendale G, Crosswell AD, et al. Yoga reduces inflammatory signaling in fatigued breast cancer survivors: A randomized controlled trial. *Psychoneuroendocrinology*. 2014;43:20-29.
4. Telles S, Naveen KV, Gaur V, Balkrishna A. Effect of one week of yoga on function and severity in rheumatoid arthritis. BMC Res Notes. 2011 Apr 12;4:118. doi: 10.1186/1756-0500-4-118.

5. Moonaz SH, Bingham CO 3rd, Wissow L, Bartlett SJ. Yoga in Sedentary Adults with Arthritis: Effects of a Randomized Controlled Pragmatic Trial. J Rheumatol. 2015 Jul;42(7):1194-202.
6. Ranjna Chawla, Bhawna Mahajan, Gaurav Thakur, Aparna, Vinod kumar Gupta, Rukamani Nair. 2015. Effect of yoga and naturopathy on physical, biochemical, immunological and inflammatory parameters in patients suffering from rheumatoid arthritis. International journal of applied ayurveda research. 2(3), 366 -375.
7. Singh VK, Bhandari RB, Rana BB. Effect of yogic package on rheumatoid arthritis. Indian J Physiol Pharmacol. 2011 Oct-Dec;55(4):329-35.

18
Yoga to Improve Mental Function

Yoga is a mind-body exercise which reduces stress, anxiety and depression and improves brain function and cognition. Cognitive functions encompass reasoning, memory, attention, and language and lead directly to the attainment of information and, thus, knowledge.

Neurocognitive disorders (NCDs) involve impairments in cognitive abilities such as memory, problem solving, and perception. It begins with delirium followed by the major NCDs, mild NCDs and their etiological subtypes.

Delirium

Delirium is a serious disturbance in mental abilities that results in confused thinking and reduced awareness of the surroundings. The start of delirium is usually rapid — within hours or a few days.

It can often be traced to one or more contributing factors, such as a severe or chronic medical illness, changes in metabolic balance (such as low sodium), medication, infection, surgery, or alcohol or drug withdrawal. Symptoms of delirium and dementia can be similar, therefore, input from a family member or caregiver is important for accurate diagnosis.

Major NCDs

Major neurocognitive disorder was previously known as dementia and the primary feature of all NCDs is an acquired cognitive decline in one or more cognitive domains. The cognitive decline must not just be a sense of a loss of cognitive abilities, but can also be observed by others like family, friends or caregivers.

Cognitive Decline in One or more Domains

- Attention
- Executive functioning
- Learning and memory
- Language
- Perceptual motor ability
- Social cognition

They interfere significantly with a person's everyday independence in major neurocognitive disorder.

Diagnosis Criteria

- Evidence of cognitive decline from previous one more domain.
- Awareness of decline by others like family, friends or caregivers
- Impairment in cognitive performance
- Cognitive deficits interfere with AD
- Not explained by a major psychiatric disorder

Ex Schizophrenia

Causation : It is specified and coded with or without behavioral disturbances

- Psychosis
- Mood disturbance
- Agitation
- Apathy
- Combativeness

Severity: Mild; Moderate, Severe

Mild Neurocognitive Disorders

Mild NCDs have cognitive deficits in the same domain as major NCDs but vary in severity. Individuals still function semi independently but needing assistance or cueing, opportunity to intervene with treatment.

Diagnostic Criteria

Mild or moderate decline in one or more cognitive domain.

- Awareness of decline by others

- Decline in performance on standardized testing
- Cognitive deficits not explained by delirium
- Deficits not explained by psychiatric disorder

Understanding causes of Major NCDs

- Frontotemporal degeneration (FTD)
- Lewy body dementia
- Vascular dementia
- Substance or medication induced
- HIV infection
- Prion disease
- Parkinson's disease dementia
- Hutington's disease dementia
- Mutiple sclerosis

Scientific Evidences of Yoga Therapy for Betterment of NCDs

Yoga and meditation may not only give a flexible body and inner peace but a combination of the two could also help improve cognitive function. In a study, led by a team of researchers from UCLA and Australia's University of Adelaide, is the first to compare yoga and meditation against memory training, which has often been considered the best way to manage mild cognitive impairment. The team followed a group of 25 participants all aged 55 and above during a three-month course of either yoga or meditation or memory training. Participants had all shown signs of mild cognitive impairment, reporting problems with their memory such as easily misplacing things, or forgetting names, faces or appointments.

Participants were split into two groups. Eleven participants attended memory enhancement training and practiced memory exercises daily, while the other 14 participants attended classes of Kundalini yoga and practiced 20 minutes of Kirtan Kriya meditation daily, which involves chanting, hand movements and visualization of light, and has already been practiced in India for hundreds of years as a way to prevent cognitive decline in older adults. All participants received brain scans and completed memory tests at both the beginning and end of the three months. The results showed that although all participants demonstrated similar improvements in verbal memory skills, the skills that are needed for remembering names, it was the participants in the group who practiced yoga and meditation that showed better improvements in visual-spatial memory skills, which help with recalling locations and navigating. In addition, participants in the yoga and meditation group also showed bigger improvements in levels of depression, anxiety, coping skills and resilience to stress, all of which are especially important when coming to terms with the onset of cognitive impairment. The study was published in the Journal of Alzheimer's Disease.

Yoga Regimen for of Neurocognitive Decline

The yoga regimen described here are extremely beneficial in prevention of **Neurocognitive diseases** (Brunner et al 2017). The practice of these yoga regimens enhances neurocognition and memory. The procedure of these yoga postures and benefits are given below:

A. Seated Asana (6-9 min)

Ardhamatsyendrasana

Procedure

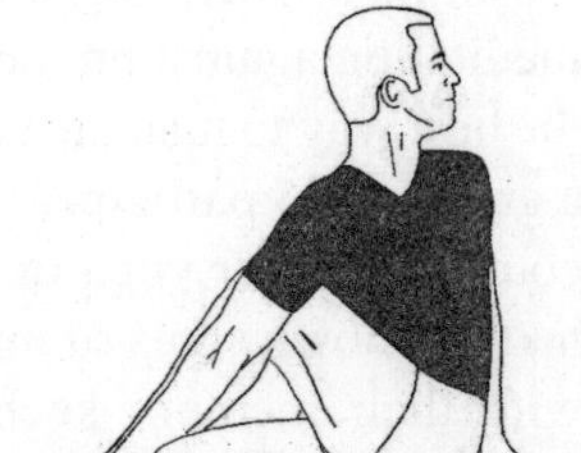

1. Sit in Vajrasana position or sit straight with stretching your legs in front of you.
2. Bend your left leg and try to touch your feet to your right buttock as shown in the image.
3. Bring your right leg outside of the left knee. Touch your feet to the ground. Keep your spine erect.
4. Exhale and turn your upper body to the right. Hold your right feet with left hand and place your right hand behind you are on the ground as shown in the image.
5. Breathe normally and hold this posture for 20 to 30 seconds. After practicing you can hold this posture for 3 to 5 minutes.
6. Now release this posture and repeat this cycle with bending right leg and bringing left leg outside of the right knee. (i.e. Twisting the opposite direction).

Benefits: It strengthens the spinal column and muscles of the back. This asana is beneficial in strengthening back muscles.

Dandasana

Procedure

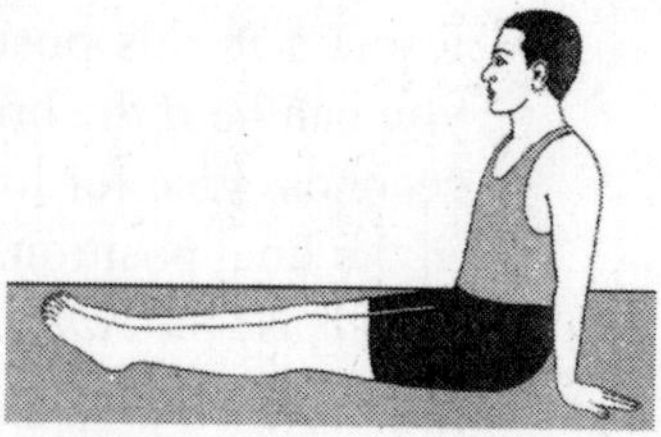

1. Sit on the ground with back straight and legs extended come in front of you. Your legs and feet ought to be hip breadth apart and parallel.
2. Press the sitting bones within the floor and pose the crown of your head to the ceiling to lengthen and straighten the spine.
3. Flexing your feet, press out through your heels.
4. Keep your palms on the ground adjacent to your hips for supporting your spine and quiet your shoulders down. Keep your body part straight however relaxed.
5. Ground your lower half firmly to the ground by relaxing the legs.
6. Hold this pose for twenty to thirty seconds.

Benefits: It helps improve posture. Strengthens back muscles. Lengthens and stretches the spine. It is beneficial for alertness and better cognition.

Janusirsasana

Procedure

1. Sit on the floor with both the legs stretched out in front of you.
2. Now bend the right leg and bring the feet close to the left thighs. Let the sole of the right foot touch the inner left thigh.
3. Adjust the right foot so that it touches the right groin.
4. Stretch the right bend leg as far back as possible without strain.
5. The left leg should remain the straight position with toes pointing upwards.
6. Take a deep breath and take your arms above the head in line with your ears.

7. Now exhale slowly and bend the body forward.
8. Let the hands go forward and grab the left foot either by the toes or the middle of the foot depending on which is more comfortable.
9. Pull your trunk forward until your forehead touches the knees.
10. Remain in this position for as long as you are comfortable. you can hold the breath if you remain in the position for few seconds. Else for longer durations, one can breathe normally in the final position.
11. To release the *Janu Sirsasana* Pose, raise your trunk to upright sitting position. Inhale while coming back to the sitting pose. Release the right leg and stretch it in front of you to come back to the starting position where both legs are stretched out in front of you.
12. Repeat this pose with the other leg, i.e. bending the left leg against the right thigh.

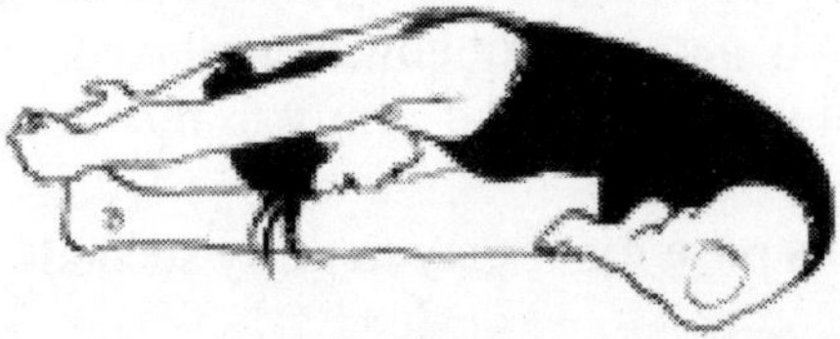

Benefits

1. *Janu Sirsasana* is an excellent asana for gaining flexibility of the legs, hamstrings, shoulders, arms and the thighs.
2. It calms the mind and has a soothing effect on the heart.

Supta Padangusthasana

Procedure

1. Lie on the floor with the legs stretched and hands relaxed on the sides.
2. Bend the right leg at the knee. Bring the knee close to the chest.
3. Hold the big toe of the right foot with the fingers. Alternatively, you can also use a strap to hold the right foot together.
4. Slowly, straighten the right leg till it is about 60 degrees to the ground. Pull the right leg further up, slowly towards you

to make it at 90 degrees to the ground. Meanwhile, keep the left leg straight, resting on the floor. With practice, one can pull the right leg further towards the head, opening up the hamstring muscles fully.

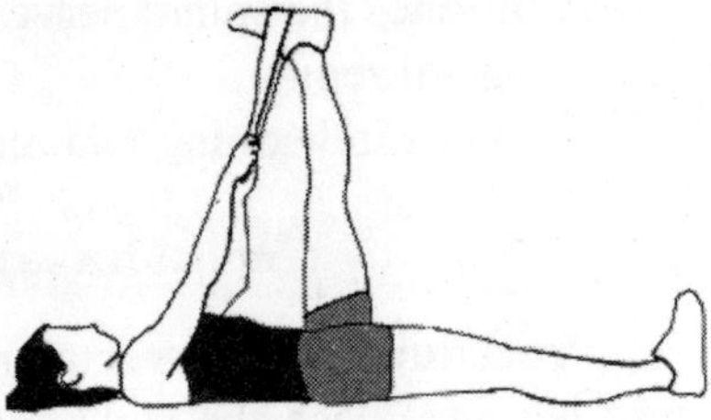

5. Breathe normally in this position and hold the big toe with the fingers (or the strap) for as long as you are comfortable.
6. To release the position, exhale and bend your right knee. Straighten out the right leg and bring it down to the floor.
7. Breathe normally and rest for few seconds and repeat the same process with the left leg.

Benefits

1. Supta Padangushtasana loosens up the hip muscles and relieves lower back pain.
2. It gives a good stretch to the hamstring muscles and makes the legs flexible.
3. Supta Padangushtasana helps to relieve sciatic pain.
4. It strengthens the cognition.

B. Standing Asana (25-27 min)

Parvatasana

Procedure

1. Straighten the leg and take it backwards. Exhale during this process. Let the right and left foot be together.
2. Raise the buttocks up. Let the two arms be on the floor and support the body weight. Lower the head to be between the two arms. The body makes the shape of a triangle when observed from the sides. It looks like a mountain and hence the name.

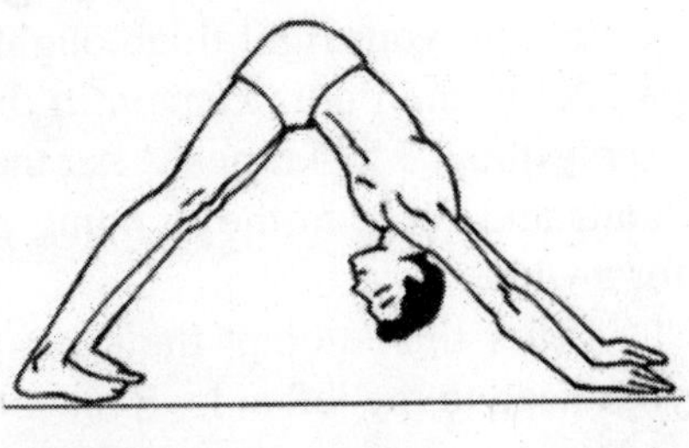

Benefits of Parvatasana

1. Parvatasana strengthens the muscles of the arms and legs.
2. It tones the spinal nerves and sends good flow of blood to the spinal region.
3. Helps in learning and memory.

Vrikshasana (Tree pose)

Procedure: Stand erects on the left leg, bend the right leg and place the right foot on the root of right thigh. Maintain the pose like as a tree on the ground. This is called vriksha-asana.

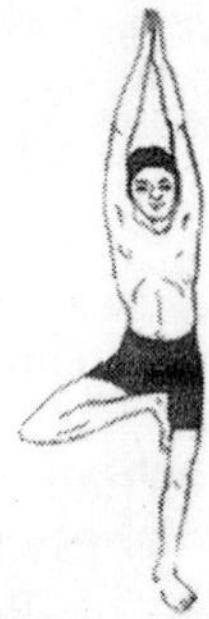

Benefits: It improves balancing skill on one foot, strengthens the muscles of the lower limbs. It is beneficial for neurocognition.

Virabhadrasana II

Procedure

First get into the standing position keep your body straight. By your legs keep a distance of 3-4 feet between each other. Breathe in and lift up your both hands. (Keep your hands parallel to the floor or ground) and turn your head to the right side. During breathing out gently turn your right feet at the angle of 90 degrees to the right side. Now gently bend your right knee little bit downward to the ground. Ensure that your right thigh ought to be parallel to the floor. Remain in this pose for 30 seconds and breathe deeply about 3 to 4 times. After that breathe out and slowly down your hands and come to the standing position and breathe normally. Rest for a while.

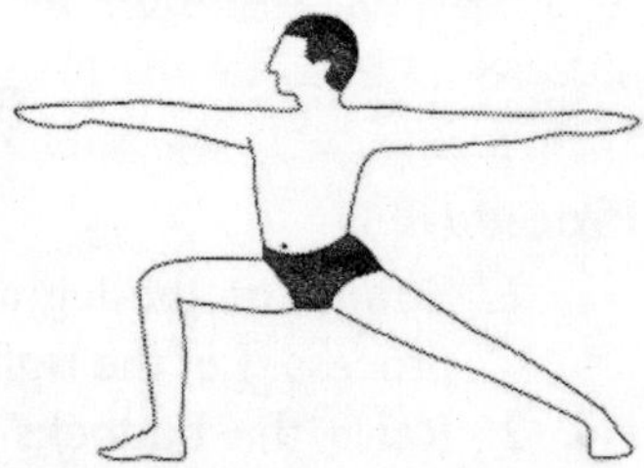

After this attempt the same steps with your left leg by turning your head to the left side. Repeat this process for 3 to 6 times.

Benefits: This Pose stretches and strengthens legs and ankles. It helps to stretch the chest, lungs and shoulders. It helps to boost the stamina. Relieves in any kind of backache. It is beneficial in the problems of cognitive decline.

Utthita Parsvakonasana

Procedure

1. *Parsvakonasana* can be started from Tadasana. Stand straight with palms of both hands facing outward and both feel adjacent to one another.
2. Exhale slowly while separating your feet until they are separated by about three feet distance.
3. Now raise your hands so that they are at the sides fully stretched and parallel to the floor. In this position, your shoulders should remain wide, the feet should be kept apart and the palms facing down.
4. Turn your left foot towards the left side, while the right foot still faces forward.
5. Turn the left thigh inwards until the ankle and the center of the left knee of your left foot are in a straight line.
6. Turn the hip slightly towards your left leg but your chest should remain straight.
7. Bend the left knee over your left ankle while inhaling, so that your shin is perpendicular to the floor.
8. The left thigh should also remain parallel to the ground with the right leg remaining straight and stretched fully from hip to ankle.
9. Now extend and stretch the right hand above your head on the left side of your body, with the palm facing the ground and remaining straight. The hand should be touching your right ear.
10. Turn your face slowly inward to look at your palm. The other hand should be touching the ankle of your left leg without taking any support from the ankle or the shoulder. The purpose of Parsvakonasana is to stretch as much towards the right side of your body as possible without feeling any discomfort.

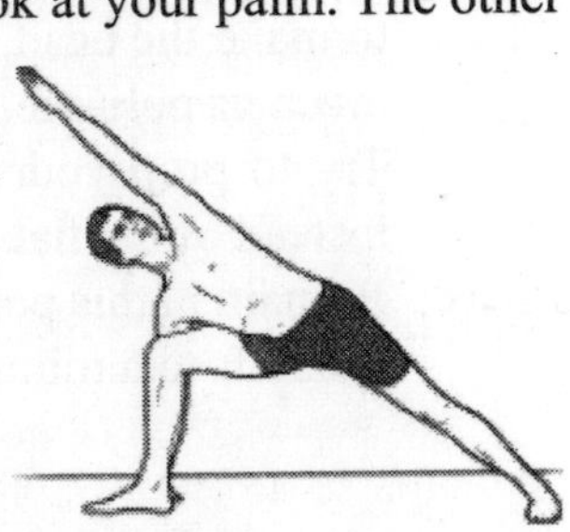

11. Push your extended hand towards the ceiling forcefully, while inhaling and exhaling. Repeat this stretching a few times and then return back to standing position.
12. Repeat the same steps with the right leg.

Benefits: It stretches out many parts, helping the legs, chest, lungs, ankles, spine, shoulders and abdomen. This pose strengthens the knees, ankles and legs while stretching muscles in the, abdomen, lungs, chest and waist. It increases stamina. It is beneficial in prevention of neurocognitive diseases.

Ardh Chandrasana

Procedure

1. Stand with legs about 3 feet apart, similar to taking the *Trikonasana*.
2. Raise both hands and bring them parallel to the ground
3. Turn the right feet towards the right making the toes point to the right side.
4. Bend to your right and bring the right hand down next to the right foot. Touch the floor with the fingers for balance.
5. Now bend the right knee till the lower leg is 90 degrees to the thighs.
6. Move further towards your right by dragging the right hand away from the right foot. Let the right palm be on the floor for support. The right leg can be slightly bent at this stage. Simultaneously raise your left leg above the floor. The left hand is pointing to the sky at this stage.
7. Now straighten the right leg and support your entire weight on your right leg as well as the right palm.
8. Make the left leg straight. Let it be parallel to the ground. The left hand remains point straight upwards towards the sky. Try to make the head, neck, trunk and left leg in a straight line as much as possible.
9. Try to prop yourself further up by balancing on the fingers instead of the flat left palm.
10. Remain in this position for as long as you are comfortable. 30 seconds to a minute is enough for beginners.

11. To release the pose, bend the right leg slightly and simultaneously bring down the left leg to the floor. Straighten the right leg and slide the right hand closer to the right foot. Raise yourself up to standing position with both hands still stretched out. Turn the right feet back to the normal front facing position.

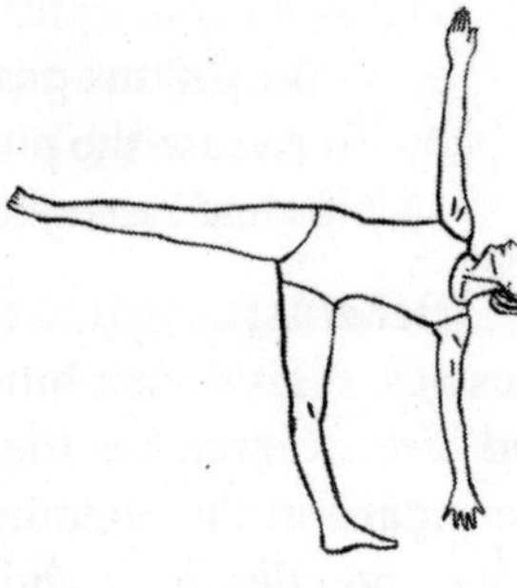

12. Repeat the same on the left side.

Benefits: It is a good pose to develop balance and coordination. It strengthens the legs, ankle, waist, abdomen, spine and arms. It can improve digestion as some parts of the abdomen are toned. It can help to release stress. It is beneficial in enhancing neuro-cognition.

Uttanasana

Procedure

1. Start in the standing position or *Tadasana*. Place the hands on the hips.
2. Take a full breath and expand your chest. Slowly exhale and fold over the hips and bend forward. Keep the torso and head in one line. At this stage the upper body will be perpendicular to the legs.
3. Now bend further and try to place the hands on the floor on the side of the legs. This requires some level of flexibility. This will loosen your hamstring muscles over a period of time. If you are not able to touch the floor with the hands, do not strain. Just go as far as you can without pain. With practice, the hamstring muscles will loosen up and you will be able to touch the floor with the hand. Make sure you do not bend the knees while performing this asana.
4. Advanced practitioners can bring the head to rest between the thighs and the hands can clasp the ankles.

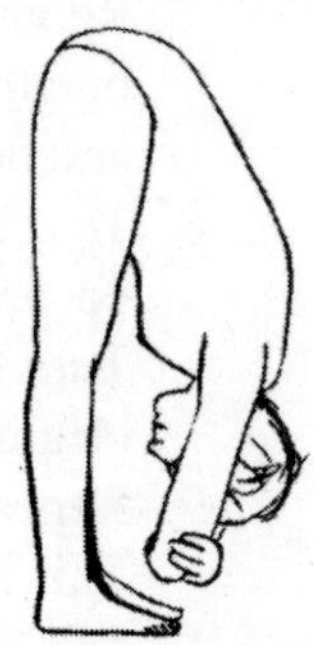

5. Maintain this position for as long as you are comfortable.
6. To release the position, inhale and bring back the hands to the hips and raise yourself up to the standing position.

Benefits: It is one of the best poses to loosen up the hamstring muscles. It gives flexibility to the hips. It removes fat around the belly and hips. It stretches the muscles of the back and the spine. It tones the organs in the abdomen and improves digestion. It relieves stress in the shoulder, back and neck muscles. It improves blood circulation and metabolism. It can give some benefits of the inverted asanas as there is more blood flow to the brain. Beneficial in improving neuro-cognition.

Virabhadrasana I

Procedure

1. Stand straight with the legs spread out. Let there be distance of at least 3 feet between the two feet.
2. Raise the hands above the head and the palms facing each other.
3. Turn to the left and slowly rotate the left foot about 90 degrees to the left so that it is aligned with the chest.
4. Turn the right foot slightly (around 15 degrees) towards the inside.
5. Bend the left knee till the thighs are parallel to the ground. The right leg should remain straight.
6. The head, the chest, the left knee and the left foot should be aligned in one direction. Now you may bring the palms closer so that they touch each other.
7. Retain this position for few breaths, which should be slow and deep.
8. To release the pose, raise yourself up and straighten the left knee. Turn to the right to go back to the original position.

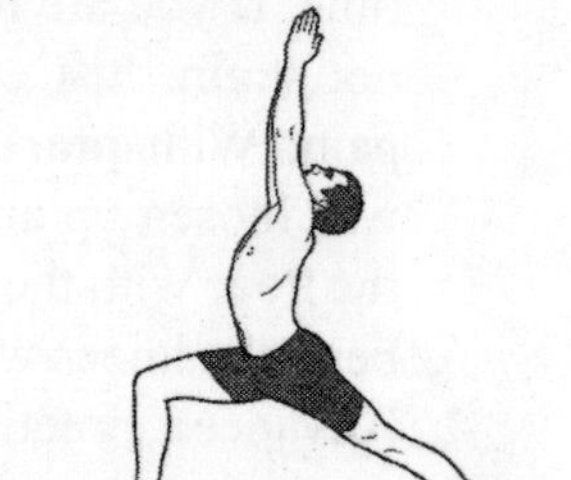

9. Repeat this on the other side too. This is done by bending the right knee and turning to the right side and aligning the head, chest, knee and foot to the right.

Benefits: It gives a good stretch to the leg muscles. It is good for the organs in the abdomen. It can improve flexibility of the back muscles. Virabhadrasana improves the nervous balance of the body. It can relieve stress in the shoulders.

Adho mukha śvānāsana

Procedure

1. Start with the kneeling position and place your palms on the floor in front of you.
2. Keep the palms spread out on the mat. The knees should be preferably behind the tail bone to get a good stretch in the final downward facing dog pose.
3. Slowly raise your knees and straighten it out. At this point the legs are straight and the weight of the body is supported by the two palms and the feet.
4. Stretch your heels and the thigh muscles while straightening the legs.
5. Tuck your belly in and push the chest slightly towards the floor while straightening the spine.
6. Make sure the heels are touching the floor. This gives a good stretch to the hamstring muscles. If your heels don't touch the floor in the initial stages, don't worry. You will definitely be able to do it after few practice sessions.
7. Place your head between the inner-side of the upper arms and look down towards the floor. This is the final pose. Breathe normally in this position. Maintain the position for as long as you are comfortable.

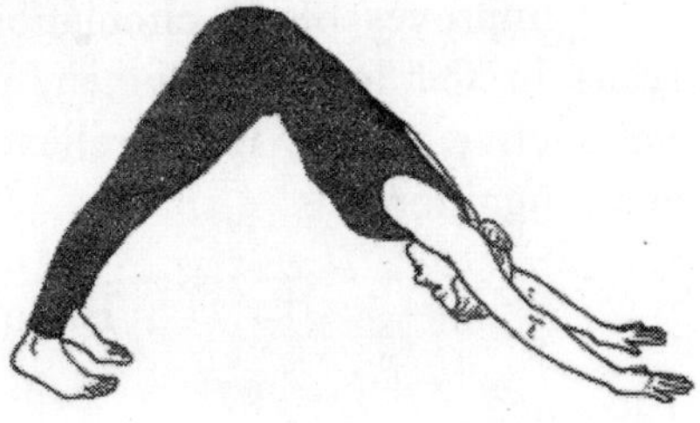

8. To release the pose, come back to the kneeling position and relax your back and arms.

Benefits: Adho Mukha Svanasana strengthens the arms and the shoulders. It can relieve anxiety and depression. It is a good relaxation pose. It relieves fatigue and relaxes the whole body.

C. Restorative Asanas (6-8 min)

Bhujangasana

Procedure

1. Lie down on your stomach on a comfortable, level surface, with your toes flat on the floor. Make your forehead rest on the ground.
2. Keep your feet together with the top portion of the feet placed against the floor. Place your palms downwards, under the shoulders - Keeping your elbows parallel and close to your torso.
3. Take a deep breath in, slowly lift your head, chest and abdomen while keeping your navel on the floor.
4. Now, pull your torso back and off the floor with the support of your hands. Breathe calmly and stay in that position for 5 to 10 breaths.

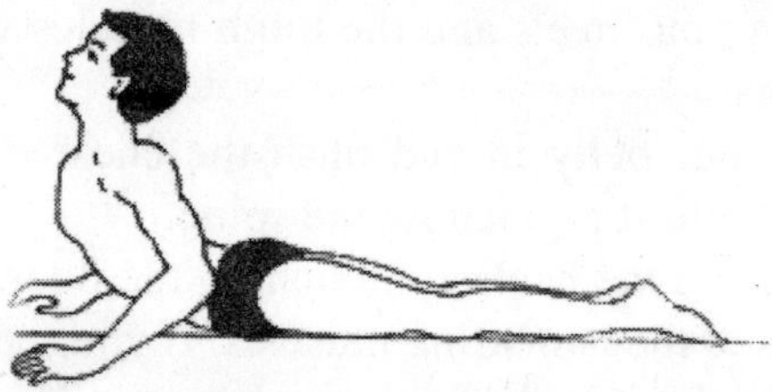

Benefits: Bhujangasana strengthens the back muscles and stretches and expands the chest.

It improves blood circulation throughout the body. Tones the organs in the lower abdomen, the digestive organs, urinary and reproductive organs. Helps relieve stress and fatigue. It helps better neuro-cognition.

Balasana

Procedure

1. Sit on your heels on a yoga mat or on the floor.
2. Either keep your knees together or apart.
3. Slowly, bend forward by lowering your forehead to touch the floor, exhaling as you do so.
4. Keep your arms alongside your body. Make sure that your palms are facing up.

5. Alternatively, you can reach out your arms towards the front of the yoga mat, palms placed facing down on the mat.
6. Now that you are in this pose, gently press your chest on the thighs (or between the thighs if the latter are apart).
7. Hold for 45 seconds to 1 minute. Regulate your breath.
9. As you inhale, imagine your breath is being driven through your navel, and pull your navel towards your spine.
10. As you exhale, soften your body and the arms. Repeat for 4-12 breaths.
11. Place your palms under the shoulders and gradually raise your upper body to return to the sitting position on the heels while inhaling. Do this very slowly as if uncurling the spine. Relax.

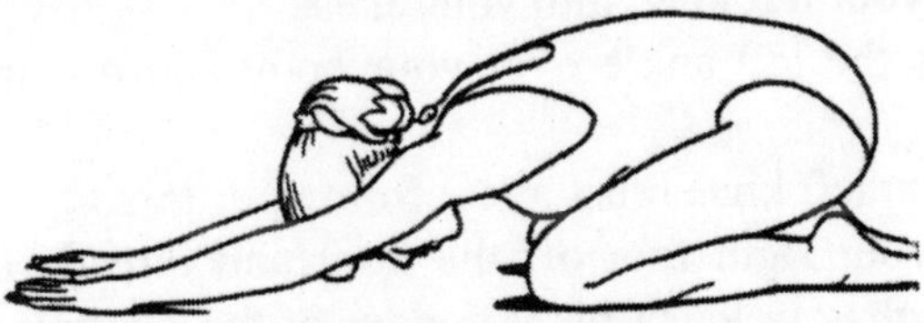

Benefits: It eases anxiety and stress. Focusing on the breathing helps relax the mind. It is beneficial in neurocognition.

Chakravakasana

Procedure

1. Come onto your hands and knees.
2. Knees should be directly underneath your hips and your hands should be directly underneath your shoulders.
3. Take a deep breath and exhale completely and slowly.
4. Slightly lift your chin.
5. When you inhale, consider that your chest should be expanded and lift it away from your belly.
6. Stretch your front body trunk front by flattening your back.
7. When you stretch your belly in, exhale.
8. Maintain this pose for some minutes.
9. Bring your chest and belly to the thighs and hips to the heels and forehead to the ground after finishing the above pose.
10. Repeat three times at the beginning.
11. Contemplate about your breathing and maintain a proper time gap.

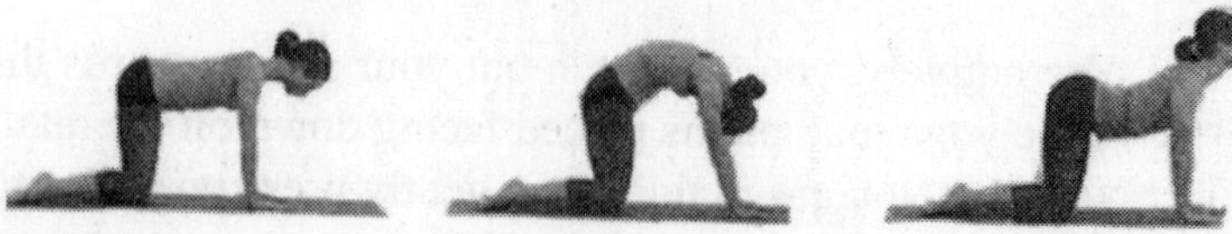

Benefits: It helps to easing the stress in the low back and gives the normal breathing flow and peace of mind. One can feel the calmness and the peace of mind. It is beneficial in neuro-cognition.

Sucirandhrasana

Procedure

1. Lie on your back with your knees bent and the soles of your feet on the floor.
2. Hug your left knee into your chest.
3. Cross the left ankle over your body and rest it on the right thigh.
4. Let the left knee relax away from your torso.
5. Lift your right foot off the floor and thread your left hand through your legs (this is the eye of the needle) so your hands meet on the back side of your right thigh. As an alternative, clasp your hands on the front side of your right shin (as shown here).
6. Using your hands, draw your right thigh toward your chest. This will cause your left hip to open.
7. Keep both feet flexed.
8. Continue to breathe deeply and relax the left knee to open the hips.
9. Repeat on the other side.

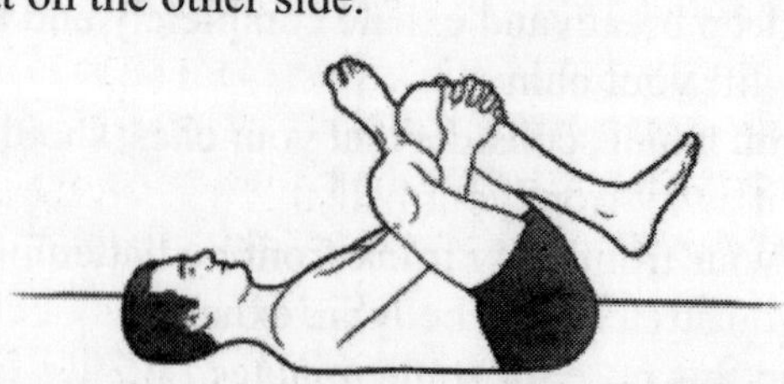

Benefits: It increases external range of motion of femur in hip socket and lengthens hip flexors (Stretches the hips). It helps in better cognition.

Viparita Karani

Procedure

1. Start with the supine position, lying on your back in a relaxed way. Let the hands rest on the floor next to the body and breathe normally.
2. Try to raise the legs slowly till the legs are almost 90 degrees to the floor.
3. Now place the hands under the lower back at the waist level. Use the hands and elbows for support to raise your body up further.
4. The breath should be held inside when you are raising the body to the vertical position
5. Use the support of the hands to raise the trunk further up, till the whole trunk is about 45 degrees to the ground and the leg are vertical. At this stage the body weight rests on the shoulders. Hands and elbows remain as props to support and balance the body.
6. In the final pose the legs are 90 degrees to the floor and the trunk is about 45 degrees to the floor.
7. Remain in this position according to your comfort. For health benefits 3-5 minutes every day is good enough. Though practitioners can go up to 15 minutes for spiritual benefits.
8. Breathe normally while maintaining the steady raised position.
9. While releasing the position, the breath is held inside and the body is slowly brought down to the supine position.
10. After performing vipareeta karani asana, usually a counter asana like matyasana, ushtrasana or supta vajrasana is performed for half the duration.

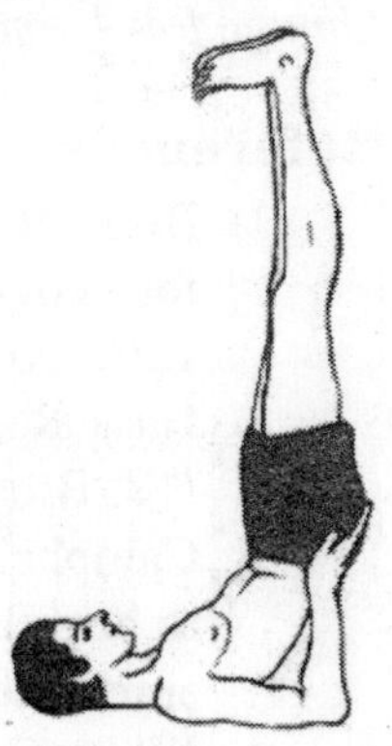

Benefits: It tones the spine, the neck, the intestines and other organs in the abdomen. It increases alertness and cognition.

D. Final relaxation: guided mindfulness meditation (10 min)
Corpse pose (supine rest)

Shavasana

Procedure

1. Lie down on back and place hands near the thighs and palm facing upwards.
2. Keep the heels slightly apart and toes pointing outwards with arelaxed body.
3. Maintain the position for 5-10 seconds or as long as comfortable.

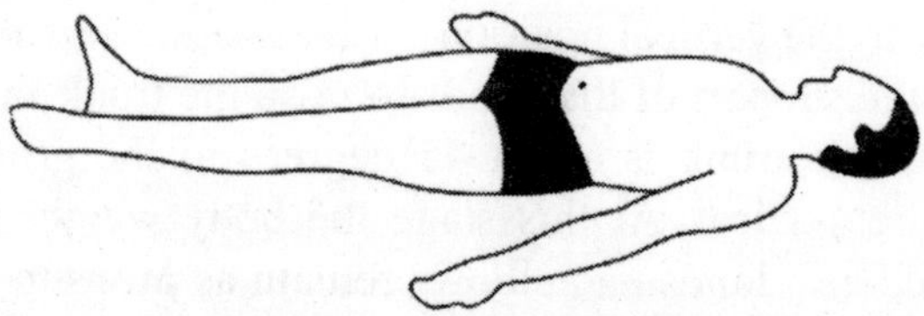

Benefits: Relaxes whole body. Relieves physical and mental fatigue. Extremely beneficial for relieving stress. Beneficial in preventing osteoporosis.

**Image for Asanas Courtesy: Google Images*

References

1. Brunner D, Abramovitch A, Etherton J. .A yoga program for cognitive enhancement. PLoS One. 2017 Aug 4; 12(8):e0182366.
2. Gass R. Chanting: Discovering Spirit in Sound. New York NY: Broadway Books, 1999.
3. Campbell D. The Mozart Effect: Tapping the power of music to heal the body, strengthen the mind, and unlock the creative spirit. New York, NY: Avon Books, 1997.
4. White G. Yoga beyond belief: Insights to awaken and deepen your practice. North Atlantic Books; 2007.
5. Stephens M. Teaching yoga: Essential foundations and techniques. North Atlantic Books; 2011 Sep 6.
6. Iyengar BK. Light on yoga: yoga dīpikā. Schocken Books; 1970.
7. Iyengar BK. BKS Iyengar yoga: The path to holistic health. Penguin; 2007 Dec 17.

❑❑❑